D1327941

Urgent Procedures in
Medical Practice

System requirement:
- Operating System – Windows Vista or above
- Recommended Web Browser – Google Chrome & Mozilla Firefox
- Essential plugins – Java & Flash player
  - Facing problems in viewing content – it may be your system does not have java enabled.
  - If Videos don't show up – it may be the system requires Flash player or need to manage flash setting. To learn more about flash setting click on the link in the help section.
  - You can test java and flash by using the links from the help section of the CD/DVD.

Accompanying CD/DVD Rom is playable only in Computer and not in DVD player.
CD/DVD has Autorun function – it may take few seconds to load on your computer. If it does not works for you then follow the steps below to access the contents manually:
- Click on my computer
- Select the **CD/DVD** drive and click open/explore – this will show list of files in the CD/DVD
- Find and double click file – "launch.html"
For more information about troubleshoot of Autorun click on:
http://support.microsoft.com/kb/330135

DISCLAIMER

The purpose of this resource is to provide a step-by-step guide to demonstrate common clinical procedures in everyday clinical practice. The description of the procedures, indications, contraindications, universal precautions and list of basic equipment are created on the basis of the most recent information from the evidence-based literature. The steps listed here are explained in limited detail and should not be performed by practitioners unfamiliar with these procedures. Healthcare providers and trainees using this video atlas and book should take all appropriate safety precautions to determine best practices for their patients in the context of the clinical situation, respecting local procedures and policies. Clinical procedures should be performed within the scope of healthcare providers' practice, in the appropriate learning environment, under the supervision of their mentors and/or supervisors, and in accordance with their governing professional association. The publisher and editor-in-chief of this book disclaim any liability, loss, injury or damage incurred as a consequence, directly or indirectly, of the use and application of any of the contents of this learning material.

Urgent Procedures in
Medical Practice

Editor-in-Chief
Sanja Kupesic Plavsic MD PhD
Professor
Department of Obstetrics and Gynecology
Associate Dean for Faculty Development
Director, Center for Advanced Teaching and Assessment in Clinical Skill
Paul L Foster School of Medicine
Texas Tech University Health Sciences Center El Paso
El Paso, Texas, USA

Technical Co-Editor
Claudia Cortez MS CTRS
Educational Unit Assistant Director
Center for Advanced Teaching and
Assessment in Clinical Skill
Paul L Foster School of Medicine
Texas Tech University Health Sciences
Center El Paso
El Paso, Texas, USA

Video Recording, Montage and Editing
Jonathan Diaz
AV Specialist
Center for Advanced Teaching and
Assessment in Clinical Skill
Paul L Foster School of Medicine
Texas Tech University Health Sciences
Center El Paso
El Paso, Texas, USA

Narration

Noel Shaheen
Medical Student
Paul L Foster School of Medicine
Texas Tech University Health Sciences
Center El Paso
El Paso, Texas, USA

Jonathan Diaz
AV Specialist
Center for Advanced Teaching and
Assessment in Clinical Skill
Paul L Foster School of Medicine
Texas Tech University Health Sciences
Center El Paso
El Paso, Texas, USA

JAYPEE

The Health Sciences Publisher
New Delhi | London | Panama

Jaypee Brothers Medical Publishers (P) Ltd

Headquarters
Jaypee Brothers Medical Publishers (P) Ltd
4838/24, Ansari Road, Daryaganj
New Delhi 110 002, India
Phone: +91-11-43574357
Fax: +91-11-43574314
Email: jaypee@jaypeebrothers.com

Overseas Offices

J.P. Medical Ltd
83 Victoria Street, London
SW1H 0HW (UK)
Phone: +44 20 3170 8910
Fax: +44 (0)20 3008 6180
Email: info@jpmedpub.com

Jaypee-Highlights Medical Publishers Inc.
City of Knowledge, Bld. 235, 2nd Floor, Clayton
Panama City, Panama
Phone: +1 507-301-0496
Fax: +1 507-301-0499
Email: cservice@jphmedical.com

Jaypee Brothers Medical Publishers (P) Ltd
17/1-B Babar Road, Block-B, Shaymali
Mohammadpur, Dhaka-1207
Bangladesh
Mobile: +08801912003485
Email: jaypeedhaka@gmail.com

Jaypee Brothers Medical Publishers (P) Ltd
Bhotahity, Kathmandu, Nepal
Phone: +977-9741283608
Email: kathmandu@jaypeebrothers.com

Website: www.jaypeebrothers.com
Website: www.jaypeedigital.com

Inquiries for bulk sales may be solicited at: jaypee@jaypeebrothers.com

Urgent Procedures in Medical Practice

First Edition: **2017**

ISBN: 978-93-5152-967-5

Printed at Sanat Printers

Dedicated to

*Our students, residents and trainees who will use
this video atlas and book to improve their clinical skills*

Contributors

Craig Ainsworth MD
Assistant Professor
Department of Internal Medicine
William Beaumont Army Medical Center
El Paso, Texas, USA

Scott Crawford MD
Assistant Professor
Department of Emergency Medicine
Paul L Foster School of Medicine
Texas Tech University Health Sciences
Center El Paso
El Paso, Texas, USA

Safa Farrag MD
Assistant Professor
Department of Internal Medicine
Paul L Foster School of Medicine
Texas Tech University Health Sciences
Center El Paso
El Paso, Texas, USA

Nicholas B Hardin DO
Resident Instructor
Radiology Department
Paul L Foster School of Medicine
Texas Tech University Health Sciences
Center El Paso
El Paso, Texas, USA

Gilberto A Gonzalez MD
Assistant Professor
Department of Orthopedic Surgery
Paul L Foster School of Medicine
Texas Tech University Health Sciences
Center El Paso
El Paso, Texas, USA

Darine Kassar MD
Assistant Professor
Neurology Department
Paul L Foster School of Medicine
Texas Tech University Health Sciences
Center El Paso
El Paso, Texas, USA

Sanja Kupesic Plavsic MD, PhD
Professor
Department of Obstetrics and
Gynecology
Associate Dean for Faculty Development
Director, Center for Advanced Teaching
and Assessment in Clinical Skill
Paul L Foster School of Medicine
Texas Tech University Health Sciences
Center El Paso
El Paso, Texas, USA

Shaked Laks MD
Assistant Professor
Radiology Department
Paul L Foster School of Medicine
Texas Tech University Health Sciences
Center El Paso
El Paso, Texas, USA

Michael F Maldonado OD
Faculty Associate
Ophthalmology Department
Paul L Foster School of Medicine
Texas Tech University Health Sciences
Center El Paso
El Paso, Texas, USA

Melissa D Mendez MD
Assistant Professor
Department of Obstetrics and
Gynecology
Paul L Foster School of Medicine
Texas Tech University Health Sciences
Center El Paso
El Paso, Texas, USA

Stacy Milan MD
Assistant Professor
Department of Surgery
Paul L Foster School of Medicine
Texas Tech University Health Sciences
Center El Paso
El Paso, Texas, USA

Benjamin R Morang DO
Resident
Department of Internal Medicine
William Beaumont Army Medical Center
El Paso, Texas, USA

Bryan Newbrough MD
Otolaryngology-Head and Neck Surgery
ENT Clinic Chief, William Beaumont
Army Medical Center
El Paso, Texas, USA

Oscar Noriega MD
Associate Professor
Family and Community Medicine
Department
Paul L Foster School of Medicine
Texas Tech University Health Sciences
Center El Paso
El Paso, Texas, USA

Victor J Olivas MD
Assistant Professor
Department of Surgery
Paul L Foster School of Medicine
Texas Tech University Health Sciences
Center El Paso
El Paso, Texas, USA

Indu Pathak MD
Assistant Professor
Pediatrics Departmen
Paul L Foster School of Medicine
Texas Tech University Health Sciences
Center El Paso
El Paso, Texas, USA

Paisith Piriyawat MD
Associate Professor
Neurology Department
Paul L Foster School of Medicine
Texas Tech University Health Sciences
Center El Paso
El Paso, Texas, USA

Carmen Prieto Jimenez MD, MPH
Assistant Professor
Pediatrics Department
Paul L Foster School of Medicine
Texas Tech University Health Sciences
Center El Paso
El Paso, Texas, USA

Gerardo Vazquez MD
Assistant Professor
Family and Community Medicine
Department
Paul L Foster School of Medicine
Texas Tech University Health Sciences
Center El Paso
El Paso, Texas, USA

Silvia Villa-Royval MD
Assistant Professor
Anesthesiology Department
Paul L Foster School of Medicine
Texas Tech University Health Sciences
Center El Paso
El Paso, Texas, USA

Preface

Video demonstrations are the most comprehensive way to learn procedures and contain information that cannot be mastered using photograph format. DVD on *Urgent Procedures in Medical Practice* presents 50 procedural skills demonstrated on partial task trainers, full body simulators, cadavers and/or on real patients in real clinical scenarios. This comprehensive video atlas contains high–yield information on core procedures in family medicine, internal medicine, emergency medicine, surgery and obstetrics and gynecology. In our DVD, 20 experienced clinicians and experts in different disciplines use clinical simulation to guide medical students, nursing students, physicians in training, junior doctors and nurses through most common procedures in clinical practice. All the videos include learning objectives, indications, contraindications, universal precautions, complications, basic equipment and step-by step guide how to prepare and execute the procedure.

In clinical practice often there is not enough time to read an article, chapter or look through a large reference when there is a patient who requires an immediate response. The accompanying book serves as a quick guide for 50 procedural skills every physician in training and practicing physician should know. Chapters featuring procedural skills provide a concise review of the procedures and include 5 multiple choice questions and answers to test the learner's knowledge. List of relevant literature sources is provided at the end of each chapter.

Combining the instructional videos and book in a practical manner allows the use of this procedure guide at the point of care as a great resource for keeping all the information at learners' fingertips. Good luck in your practice!

Sanja Kupesic Plavsic

Acknowledgments

First and foremost, I want to express my gratitude to my collaborators, Claudia and Jonathan for devoting their time, knowledge, skills and creativity in this project. I thank each of the contributors for sharing their expertise in procedural skills. Special thanks to Dr Lisa Montgomery who proposed and initiated this publication, and to my colleagues, collaborators, residents and students who provide continued sources of encouragement and inspiration.

I also wish to thank the dedicated staff of M/s Jaypee Brothers Medical Publishers (P) Ltd, New Delhi, India, who adopted new challenges and encouraged me to complete this innovative step-by-step guide to procedural skills. The team has always provided excellent technical support.

I would like to acknowledge and thank the Willed Body Program at TTUHSC El Paso Paul L Foster School of Medicine for collaboration in this educational project. Last but not least, I want to thank the Center for Advanced Teaching and Assessment in Clinical Simulation (ATACS) staff for providing a great and inspiring environment for video recording. This would not have been possible without their continuous support!

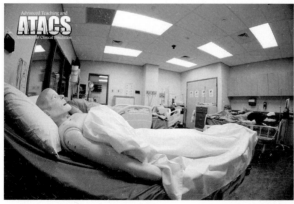
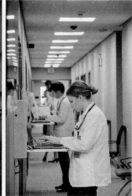

Contents

DVD Contents

Skin Adhesives

Pathak I

OBJECTIVES

- Know gluing technique
- List the indications for skin adhesives
- Know the complications of skin adhesives
- Know how to perform skin gluing

INTRODUCTION/BACKGROUND

- Dermabond is a cyanoacrylate adhesive: Combines cyanoacetate and formaldehyde with a base to form a liquid
  - Forms a cyanoacrylate bridge with the skin's moisture, binding the wound edges together
  - Is a flexible water-resistant protective coating
  - Healing occurs below skin level
  - No need for adhesive removal
  - Meant to replace sutures 5-0 or smaller
- Advantages over sutures
  - Maximum strength at 2½ minutes
  - Equivalent in strength to healed tissue at seven days post-repair
  - Can be applied using only a topical anesthetic, no needles
  - Water-resistant covering
  - Does not require removal of sutures.

UNIVERSAL PRECAUTIONS

- Gloves must be worn
- Evaluate the need for face and eye protection as well as a gown
- Only the necessary amount of adhesive should be used
- Excess adhesive must be quickly removed.

OBTAIN INFORMED CONSENT

- Introduce yourself to the patient
- Explain the procedure to the patient and gain informed consent to continue
- Explain that the adhesive may produce a sensation of heat while drying.

INDICATIONS

- Properly selected wounds on the face, extremities and torso may be closed up to the discretion of the physician
- Extremity and torso wounds tend to heal better when subcutaneous sutures are placed first
- If areas of high tension or mobility, splint to prevent premature peeling
- No need for follow-up.

CONTRAINDICATIONS

- Jagged or stellate lacerations
- Bites, punctures or crush wounds
- Contaminated wounds
- Mucosal surfaces
- Axillae and perineum (high-moisture areas)
- Hands, feet and joints (unless kept dry and immobilized).

COMPLICATIONS

- Immediate complications
  - Hematoma formation
  - Wound infection
  - Excess adhesive
  - Edges misaligned
  - Glued eyelids
- Late complications
  - Dehiscence
  - Scar formation.

BASIC EQUIPMENT

- Gauze
- Vial of dermabond
- Antiseptic
- Topical anesthetic.

PREPARATION

- Ensure wound irrigation and cleansing
- Clean smaller lacerations with antibacterial and flush with sterile saline solution
- Deeper wounds should undergo these same steps but may also require subcutaneous sutures to strengthen the wound closure.

PROCEDURE STEPS

- Apply topical anesthetic as needed
- Prepare wound with antiseptic
- Appose wound edges
- Crush Dermabond vial and invert
- Gently brush adhesive over laceration
- Avoid pushing adhesive into wound
- Apply three layers of adhesive
- No covering is needed
- No removal necessary.

SELF-ASSESSMENT QUIZ

1. What is an appropriate adhesive site?
   a. Elbow   b. Knuckle
   c. Labia   d. Scalp
2. What does the adhesive use to bond to the skin?
   a. Skin moisture   b. Saline
   c. Antiseptic   d. Anesthetic
3. Which of the following is not an indication for skin adhesion?
   a. Wound with minimal tension   b. Moist location of wound
   c. Edges that are easily approximated d. Smooth edged wound
4. How is skin adhesive removed when the eyelid is glued shut?
   a. Force eyelids open
   b. Warm the eyelids and it will release in 2 hours
   c. Apply ointment and it will release in 3 days
   d. Take the patient to surgery and cut the eyelid open
5. To what wound depth should the adhesive be applied?
   a. Surface only   b. 2 cm below surface
   c. 5 cm below surface   d. Full depth of laceration

Answers

1. d   2. a   3. b   4. c   5. a

SUGGESTED READING

1. Bruns TB, Robinson BS, Smith RJ, et al. A new tissue adhesive for laceration repair in children. J Pediatr. 1998;132:1067-70.
2. Bruns TB, Simon HK, McLario DJ, Sullivan KM, Wood RJ, Anand KJ. Laceration repair using a tissue adhesive in a children's emergency department. Pediatrics. 1996;98:673-5.
3. Edlich RF: Tissue adhesives—revisited. Ann Emerg Med. 1998;31:106-7.
4. Quinn J, Wells G, Sutcliffe T. et al. Tissue adhesive versus suture wound repair at 1 year: Randomized clinical trial correlating early, 3-month, and 1-year cosmetic outcome. Ann Emerg Med. 1998;32:645-9.
5. Quinn JV, Drzewiecki A, Li MM, Stiell IG, Sutcliffe T, Elmslie TJ, et al. A randomized, controlled trial comparing a tissue adhesive with suturing in the repair of pediatric facial lacerations. Ann Emerg Med. 1993;22:1130-5.
6. Quinn JV, Wells GA. An assessment of clinical wound evaluation scales. Acad Emerg Med. 1998;5:583-6.
7. Simon HK, McLario DJ, Bruns TB, Zempsky WT, Wood RJ, Sullivan KM. Long-term appearance of lacerations repaired using a tissue adhesive. Pediatrics. 1997;99:193-5.
8. Singer AJ, Hollander JE, Valentine SM, Thode HC Jr, Henry MC. Association of training level and short-term cosmetic appearance of repaired lacerations. Acad Emerg Med. 1996;3:378-83.
9. Singer AJ, Hollander JE, Valentine SM, Turque TW, McCuskey CF, Quinn JV. Prospective, randomized, controlled trial of tissue adhesive (2-octylcyanoacrylate) vs. standard wound closure techniques for laceration repair. Acad Emerg Med. 1998;5:94-9.
10. Toriumi DM, O'Grady K, Desai D, Bagal A. Use of octyl-2-cyanoacrylate for skin closure in facial plastic surgery. Plast Reconstr Surg. 1998;102:2209-19.

Skin Stapling

Milan S

OBJECTIVES

- Know skin stapling techniques
- List the indications for skin stapling
- Know the complications of skin stapling
- Know how to perform skin stapling

INTRODUCTION/BACKGROUND

- Three phases of wound healing
  - Inflammation
  - Tissue formation
  - Tissue remodeling
- Primary intention
  - Decreased dead space minimizes scar tissue
- Secondary intention
  - Wound is left to heal spontaneously
- Skin stapler is like an office stapler except
  - It staples patient's wounds
  - Stapler is nonrefillable
  - Staple is of inert metal and does not rust
- Staples as compared to sutures
  - Are faster, have lower infection rates
  - Less crushing to tissues
  - Staples are nonreactive with tissues.

UNIVERSAL PRECAUTIONS

- Gloves must be worn while stapling
- Evaluate the need for face and eye protection, as well as a gown
- Staples should go into the patient
- Staples that misfire or must be removed should be placed into an appropriate sharps container.

OBTAIN INFORMED CONSENT

- Introduce yourself to the patient
- Explain the procedure to the patient and gain informed consent to continue
- Explain that the staples produce a pinching sensation that is quickly over

INDICATIONS

- Wound with minimal tension
  - Scalp, extremities or torso
  - Clean edges that are easily approximated
- Need for quick repair
  - Mass casualty or multiple trauma situations
  - Pediatric lacerations.

CONTRAINDICATIONS

- Staples are metal
  - Cannot be placed prior to CT or MRI
- Not for use on
  - Deep wounds
  - Face, hands or feet
  - Inadequate hemostasis
  - When less than 5 mm of tissue exists between the stapled skin and vital underlying structures.

COMPLICATIONS

- Immediate complications
  - Hematoma formation
  - Wound infection
- Late complications include scar formation
  - Excess tension
  - Lack of eversion
- Allergic response to stainless steel
  - Chromium, nickel, copper, cobalt, iron.

BASIC EQUIPMENT

- Gauze
- Surgical scrub brush
- Normal saline
- Antimicrobial skin cleanser (e.g. Hibiclens)
- Lidocaine
- Stapling device
- Tweezers

PREPARATION

- Mechanical cleansing
  - Surgical scrub brush, soap and water
  - Normal saline irrigation
- Chemical cleansing
  - Betadine, Hibiclens
  - Freshen wound edges
  - Anesthetic
  - Lidocaine 1% +/– epinephrine.

PROCEDURE STEPS

- Approximate and evert skin edges
- Line up center of staple over the skin
- Place on skin with downward pressure
- Squeeze the trigger firmly and completely
- Relax thumb pressure to release
- Repeat along the incision.

REMOVAL

- Ensure staples are not rotated
- Place the lower jaw of the remover under the staple
- Lift slightly to straighten the staple
- Gently squeeze the handles together
- Lift the staple straight up and remove.

SELF-ASSESSMENT QUIZ

1. What is an appropriate stapling site?
   - a. Face
   - b. Hands
   - c. Scalp
   - d. Toes
2. What is one difference between an office stapler and a skin stapler?
   - a. Skin stapler is refillable
   - b. Skin staple is of inert metal
   - c. Office staple will not rust
   - d. Office stapler is nonrefillable
3. Which of the following is not an indication for skin stapling?
   - a. Wound with minimal tension
   - b. Edges that are easily approximated
   - c. Need for quick repair
   - d. None of the above
4. An allergy to which of the following would be a contraindication to skin stapling?
   - a. Stainless steel
   - b. Platinum
   - c. Gold
   - d. Silver
5. What wound depth would be appropriate for stapler repair?
   - a. 6 cm without underlying vital tissue
   - b. 3 cm with underlying vital tissue
   - c. 5 mm without underlying vital tissue
   - d. 3 mm with underlying vital tissue

Answers

1. c   2. b   3. d   4. a   5. c

SUGGESTED READING

1. Gatt D, Quick CRG, Owen-Smith MS. Staples for wound closure: a controlled trial. Ann R Coll Surg Engl. 1985;67:318-20.
2. James, D. Skin stapling. In: Procedures for Primary Care, 3rd Ed. Philadelphia, USA: Elsevier Mosby. 2011. p. 235-7.
3. Johnson A, Rodeheaver GT, Durand LS, Edgerton MT, Edlich RF. Automatic disposable stapling devices for wound closure. Ann Emerg Med. 1981;10:631-5.
4. Meiring L, Cilliers K, Barry R, Nel CJC. A comparison of a disposable skin stapler and nylon sutures for wound closure. SAfr Med J. 1982;62:371-2.
5. Pickford IR, Brennan SS, Evans M, Pollock AV. Two methods of skin closure in abdominal operations: A controlled clinical trial. Br J Surg. 1983;70(4):226-8.
6. Ranaboldo CJ, Rowe-Jones DC. Closure of laparotomy wounds: Skin staples versus sutures. Br J Surg. 1992;72:1172-3.
7. Reiter D. Methods and materials for wound closure. Otolaryngol Clin North Am. 1995;28(5):1069-80.
8. Singer AJ, Clark RA. Cutaneous wound healing. N Engl J Med. 1999;341(10):738-46.
9. Stillman RM, Bella FJ, Seligman SJ. Skin wound closure: The effect of various wound closure methods on susceptibility to infection. Arch Surg. 1980;115:674-5.
10. Stillman RM, Marino CA, Seligman SJ. Skin staples in potentially contaminated wounds. Arch Surg. 1984;119:821-2.
11. Thomsen TW, Barclay DA, Setnik GS. Basic laceration repair. New Eng J Med. 2006;355(e18).

Suturing Skin Lacerations

Milan S

OBJECTIVES

- Describe suturing skin laceration technique
- List the indications for suturing of skin lacerations
- Describe the different types of suture material and their unique properties
- List the complications of suturing skin lacerations
- Know how to perform skin suturing

INTRODUCTION

- Suturing is the joining of tissues with needle and suture so that the tissues bind together and heal
- The suture technique varies based on location of wound and tension across the laceration
- The correct stitch with the correct type of suture is important to achieve optimal wound healing.

UNIVERSAL PRECAUTIONS

- Gloves must be worn
- Evaluate the need for face and eye protection as well as a gown.

OBTAIN INFORMED CONSENT

- Introduce yourself to the patient
- Explain the procedure to the patient and gain informed consent to continue
- Explain that there may be some transient discomfort with the administration of the local anesthesia.

INDICATIONS

- Suturing can be performed on any skin laceration or wound needing closure
- As compared to other closure techniques suturing
  - Is the best choice in areas of high tension
  - Best choice over joints
  - Best choice in deep wounds
  - Best choice in areas of high moisture.

CONTRAINDICATIONS

- Extended interval between injury and repair
- Consider other factors including:
  - Patient's age and state of health
  - Potential for foreign bodies embedded in the wound
  - Associated injuries to underlying structures
  - Degree of contamination.

COMPLICATIONS

- Immediate complications
  - Hematoma formation
  - Wound infection
- Late complications
  - Scar formation.

BASIC EQUIPMENT

- Sutures
- Needle driver
- Toothed forceps
- Suture scissors
- Antiseptic
- Lidocaine—maximum dose is 4 mg/kg
- Wound dressings, tape
- Consider need for tetanus immunization
  - Primary course: Three doses of tetanus vaccine with a booster every 10 years
    - Course incomplete: Tetanus immune globulin, and tetanus-diphtheria (Td) or tetanus toxoid, and schedule to complete vaccinations
  - Booster <5 years: No treatment
  - Booster >5 years:
    - Clean wound: Td or tetanus toxoid
    - Dirty wound: Immune globulin and Td or tetanus toxoid.

TYPES OF SUTURES

- Natural materials are more traditional
  - Gut, cotton, silk
- Synthetic materials cause less reaction
  - All sutures other than gut, cotton and silk
- Monofilament sutures
  - Less drag, susceptible to damage, less risk of infection over multifilament
- Absorbable: Quick-healing wounds, give minimal support
  - Monofilament: Monocryl, Maxon, and PDS
  - Multifilament: Vicryl and Dexon
- Nonabsorbable: Longer support
  - Monofilaments: Prolene, Novafil, PTFE
  - Multifilament: Polyester
  - Available as either: Nylon or steel.

SITES

- Face: 1% lidocaine with epinephrine
  - 4.0 or 5.0 nonabsorbable monofilament
  - 5.0 absorbable monofilament on cutting needle
  - Interrupted or intracuticular technique. Sutures out in 3–5 days
- Scalp: 1% lidocaine with epinephrine
  - 2 or 3.0 nonabsorbable monofilament on a cutting needle
  - Interrupted or mattress. Remove in 10 days.
- Ear: 1% or 2% plain lidocaine, or field block
  - 1.0 synthetic absorbable on taper needle for perichondrium
  - 1.0 synthetic nonabsorbable monofilament on cutting needle for skin
  - Interrupted sutures. Sutures out in 5 days.
- Lip: 1 or 2% lidocaine with epinephrine consider block
  - 4.0 or 5.0 synthetic absorbable on taper needle for deeper layers
  - 1.0 synthetic monofilament on cutting needle for skin
  - Interrupted sutures, remove in 3–5 days
- Oral cavity: 1 or 2% lidocaine with epinephrine
  - 4.0 absorbable gut or synthetic on taper needle, mattress technique
  - Remove any remaining after 7 days
- Hands and feet: 1% plain lidocaine, or consider regional block with bupivacaine
  - 1.0 or 5.0 nonabsorbable synthetic monofilament on cutting needle
  - Interrupted or running sutures. Remove in 10–14 days
- Nail beds: 2% plain lidocaine, or consider regional block with bupivacaine
  - 5.0 plain gut on taper needle. Use a stent for the nail fold
  - Interrupted sutures. Allow to absorb.

- Torso: 1% lidocaine with epinephrine
  - 4.0 or 5.0 nonabsorbable synthetic monofilament on cutting needle
  - Interrupted or running sutures. Remove in 10 days
- Extremity: 1 or 2% lidocaine with epinephrine
  - 1.0 or 4.0 absorbable synthetic on taper needle for muscle or fascia; interrupted
  - 5.0 nonabsorbable monofilament on cutting needle for skin; interrupted or running sutures
  - Remove in 10 days.

PREPARATION

- Wounds in need of the operating room
  - Excessive length or depth, potentially requiring general anesthesia
  - Severe contamination requiring extensive cleansing or debridement
  - Open fractures, tendon, nerve, or major blood vessel injury
  - Complex structures requiring meticulous repair (eyelid)
- Ensure wound irrigation and cleansing
  - Mechanical cleansing: Surgical scrub brush, soap and water
  - Mechanical cleansing: Normal saline irrigation using a 30 cc or 60 cc syringe with an 18 or 20 gauge needle to develop pressure. Use 100 cc of saline for each cm of wound
  - Chemical cleansing: Betadine, Savlon, or Hibiclens
  - Freshen wound edges with scalpel or scissors
- Sharp undermining of the tissues may be needed to minimize wound tension:
  - Accomplish this by using a scalpel or scissors in the subdermal plane
  - Additionally, achieve hemostasis prior to wound closure to avoid future complications such as hematoma
  - Use atraumatic skin-handling technique with skin hooks and small forceps
- Deep sutures may need to be placed using absorbable sutures
  - Eliminate dead space and relieve tension
  - Ensure proper alignment of the edges
  - Contribute to the wound's final eversion
- Good approximation of wound edges
  - Wound edges are not only aligned but are also everted to avoid unnecessary depression of the resultant scar.

PROCEDURE STEPS

- Simple interrupted: To close dead space
  - Insert the needle at a 90° angle to the skin within 1–2 mm of the wound edge and in the superficial layer

- – Needle through directly opposite and equidistant to the initial insertion
- – Oppose equal amounts of tissue on each side
- – A surgeon's knot secures each suture
- – Place all knots on the same side
- Simple running suture
  - – Similar to the simple suture without a knotted completion after each throw
  - – Quicker, but if too tight can cause excess tension and strangulation at the suture line
  - – Simple locked running suture allows for greater accuracy in skin alignment, with the same advantages and similar risks
  - – Easy to remove, more watertight than simple sutures
- Vertical mattress aids in everting the skin edges, and use for attachment to fascial layer
  - – The needle is inserted at 90° to the skin surface near the wound edge and through deeper layers
  - – Exit through the opposite wound edge at the same level, and then turn it to repenetrate that same edge, more distant from the edge
  - – Final exit is through the opposing skin edge, at a greater distance than the original site
  - – Place the knot at the surface
- Horizontal mattress: To oppose skin of different thickness
  - – Entrance and exit sites for the needle are at the same distance from the wound edge. Half-buried mattress sutures are useful at corners.
  - – On one side, an intradermal component is placed (the surface is not penetrated)
  - – Place the knot at the skin surface on the opposing edge of the wound
- Subcuticular sutures: Do not penetrate the skin surface
  - – Sutures can be placed intradermally in either a simple or running fashion
  - – Place the needle horizontally in the dermis, 1–2 mm from the wound edge
  - – The knot is buried in the simple suture, allows for minimal tension on the edge
  - – In a continuous subcuticular stitch, the suture ends can be taped to the skin surface without knotting.

REMOVAL

- In general, remove nonabsorbable suture after 4–5 days
- In certain situations, nonabsorbable suture can be removed at 10–12 days

SELF-ASSESSMENT QUIZ

1. Which wound does not require repair in the OR?
   a. Excessive length
   b. Severe contamination
   c. Clean wound
   d. Open fracture
2. Which is not a contraindication for suturing?
   a. 15 hours past injury
   b. 15 hours past facial injury
   c. Contaminated wounds
   d. Stable health
3. What is the best stitch to use on the lip?
   a. Simple running stitch
   b. Mattress
   c. Interrupted stitch
   d. Subcuticular
4. When are nonabsorbable sutures preferred to absorbable?
   a. Low tension
   b. Slow-healing wounds
   c. No need for support
   d. Quick-healing wounds
5. Which is the incorrect stitch use combination?
   a. Horizontal mattress: Skin of different thicknesses
   b. Vertical mattress: Attachment to fascia
   c. Simple running stitch: Superficial wound
   d. Subcuticular: Superficial wound

Answers

1. c   2. b   3. c   4. b   5. d

SUGGESTED READING

1. Diwan R, Tromovitch TA, Glogau RG, Stegman SJ. Secondary intention healing. The primary approach for management of selected wounds. Arch Otolaryngol Head Neck Surg. 1989;115(10):1248-9.
2. Kanzler MH, Gorsulowsky DC, Swanson NA. Basic mechanisms in the healing cutaneous wound. J Dermatol Surg Oncol 1986;12(11):1156-64.
3. Kuo F, Lee D, Rogers GS. Prospective, randomized, blinded study of a new wound closure film versus cutaneous suture for surgical wound closure. Dermatol Surg. 2006;32(5):676-81.
4. Moy RL, Waldman B, Hein DW. A review of sutures and suturing techniques. J Dermatol Surg Oncol. 1992;18(9):785-95.
5. Pickford IR, Brennan SS, Evans M, Pollock AV. Two methods of skin closure in abdominal operations: A controlled clinical trial. Br J Surg 1983;70(4):226-8.
6. Reiter D. Methods and materials for wound closure. Otolaryngol Clin North Am. 1995;28(5):1069-80.
7. Reynolds RD. Laceration and incision repair: Suture tying. In Procedures for Primary Care, 3rd Ed. Philadelphia, USA: Elsevier Mosby. 2011:179-83.
8. Scott M. 32,000 years of sutures. NATNEWS. 1983;20(5):15-7.
9. Singer AJ, Clark RA. Cutaneous wound healing. N Engl J Med 1999;341(10):738-46.
10. Spotnitz WD, Falstrom JK, Rodeheaver GT. The role of sutures and fibrin sealant in wound healing. Surg Clin North Am. 1997;77(3):651-69.
11. Zempsky WT, Zehrer CL, Lyle CT, Hedbloom EC. Economic comparison of methods of wound closure: Wound closure strips vs. sutures and wound adhesives. Int Wound J. 2005;2(3):272-81.

Nail Removal

Crawford S

OBJECTIVES

- Describe nail removal technique
- List the indications for nail removal
- Describe the complications of nail removal
- Know how to perform nail removal
- Know how to perform nail bed trephination

INTRODUCTION/BACKGROUND

- Nails have a function
  - Protect digit tip, contribute to sensation, involved in peripheral circulation
- Abnormal nails can cause pain
- In nail trauma, also assess digit,
  - Evaluate for tendon injury by assessing digital movement
  - Assess sensation of each aspect of digit
  - If fracture suspected, evaluate with X-ray.

UNIVERSAL PRECAUTIONS

- Gloves must be worn while performing procedure
- Evaluate the need for face and eye protection.

OBTAIN INFORMED CONSENT

- Introduce yourself to the patient
- Explain the procedure to the patient, as well as the risks and benefits
- Gain informed consent to continue.

INDICATIONS

- Nail deformities
  - Curved nail: Onychogryposis
  - Ingrown nail: Onychocryptosis
  - Fungal infection: Onychomycosis
- Nail bed laceration
- Extensive paronychia (nail fold infection)
- Complex nail injury.

CONTRAINDICATIONS

- Bleeding diathesis
- If allergic to local anesthetic, do not use the anesthetic.

COMPLICATIONS

- Bleeding
- Infection
- Anatomical nail injury
  - Skin at the nail sides are the perionychium
  - Eponychium is skin proximal to the nail
  - Germinal matrix lies under eponychium and is the source of the nail's growth
  - Nail matrix is under the nail and adheres the nail to the digit.

BASIC EQUIPMENT

- Betadine
- Sterile towels
- Syringe and needle
- Local anesthetic without epinephrine
- Finger tourniquet
- Scissors or nail elevator
- Hemostats
- Antibiotic ointment, gauze and dressing.

PREPARATION

- Clean digit with betadine
- Place extremity in a comfortable position that allows your access to the nail
- Perform digital block
  - The palmar/plantar nerves innervate the palmar/plantar surface and the nail bed
  - Dorsal nerve innervates dorsum of the digit
  - Perform block as described in separate anesthetic procedure.

PROCEDURE STEPS

- Place tourniquet at base of digit
- Instrument beneath the following areas:
  - Free edge of the nail: Advance between the nail plate and nail bed until reach the nail fold
  - Under eponychium, freeing it from the nail
- Avulse nail: Grasp with hemostat and pull nail straight out with firm, steady traction
- Remove tourniquet. Apply antibiotic ointment, gauze and dressing.

INGROWN TOENAIL REMOVAL

- Onychocryptosis: Lateral nail hypertrophy
- Removal procedure is adjusted so only the lateral edge of the nail is freed
  - Use scissors to cut proximally to ingrown edge, making a smooth new edge
  - Perform lateral nail avulsion by grasping and removing the free lateral nail with hemostat
- Consider ablation of lateral nail bed with electric or phenol cauterization.

SUBUNGUAL HEMATOMA TREPHINATION

- Highly vascular nail bed can bleed, causing increased pressure under the nail
- Drainage does not accelerate healing or prevent infection
- Nail bed trephination is indicated within 48 hours of injury, when nail edges are intact and subungual hematoma is painful
  - Any hematoma size can be drained if edges are intact. Consider digital block for pain
- Contraindicated in patients with nail-bed lacerations or distal phalangeal tuft fracture
- Complications
  - Injury to nail bed if tool advanced too far
  - Infection if nail not clean before procedure
  - Ineffective drainage if hole is too small
- Equipment includes betadine, gauze, topical antibiotic and puncture tool
  - 18 G (gauge) needle, electrocautery tool or paper clip
- Procedure
  - Prepare the nail with betadine
  - Tool preparation
    - Paperclip: Heat end in open flame to sterilize
    - Activate cautery so that tip is hot, then use
    - 18 G needle: Twirl needle with applying pressure

– Make a hole at the base of the nail or in the center of the hematoma, applying pressure to get fluid to drain out until nail bed returns back to normal color

– Apply antibacterial ointment and gauze.

SELF-ASSESSMENT QUIZ

1. What is the location of the perionychium?
   a. Skin at the nail sides
   b. Skin proximal to the nail
   c. Under the eponychium
   d. Under the nail
2. When is nail bed trephination indicated?
   a. Within 48 hours of injury
   b. Nail edges are intact
   c. Subungual hematoma is painful
   d. All of the above
3. What is not an indication for nail removal?
   a. Nail deformities
   b. Nail bed laceration
   c. Extensive paronychia
   d. Subungual hematoma
4. What should be assessed in every nail trauma?
   a. Digital flexion
   b. Digital extension
   c. Digital X-ray
   d. Capillary refill
5. Which is not a major function of a nail?
   a. Protect digit tip
   b. Aid in scratching
   c. Contribute to sensation
   d. Involved in peripheral circulation

Answers

1. a   2. d   3. d   4. c   5. b.

SUGGESTED READING

1. Batrick N, Hashemi K, Freij R. Treatment of uncomplicated subungual haematoma. Emerg Med J. 2003;20:65.
2. Denkler K. A comprehensive review of epinephrine in the finger: To do or not to do. Plast Reconstr Surg. 2001;108:114.
3. Jellinek NJ, Bauer JH. En bloc excision of the nail. Dermatol Surg. 2010;36:1445.
4. Jellinek NJ. Nail surgery: Practical tips and treatment options. Dermatol Ther. 2007;20:68.
5. Moossavi M, Scher RK. Complications of nail surgery: A review of the literature. Dermatol Surg. 2001;27:225.
6. Quill G, Myerson M. A guide to office treatment on ingrown toenails. Hosp Med. 1994;30:51-4.
7. Richert B, Haneke E, Di Chiacchio N. Surgery of the nail bed. Nail Surgery. Informa Healthcare, New York; 2011. p. 55.
8. Zook EG, Guy RJ, Russell RC. A study of nail bed injuries: Causes, treatment, and prognosis. J Hand Surg Am. 1984;9:247.
9. Zuber TJ, Pfenninger JL. Management of ingrown toenails. Am Fam Physician. 1995;52:181-90.

Wart, Corn and Callus Removal

Olivas VJ

OBJECTIVES

- Describe warts, corn and callus removal technique
- List the indications for wart, corn and callus removal
- Describe the complications of wart, corn and callus removal
- Know how to perform the techniques of wart, corn and callus removal

INTRODUCTION/BACKGROUND

- Corns, calluses and warts are all forms of hyperkeratosis
  - Cutaneous warts are benign proliferations of skin caused by HPV infection
  - Corns are lesions with a central core of keratin from mechanical stressors at pressure points causing friction on skin
  - Callouses are diffuse thickening of stratum corneum from friction on the skin (without a central core).

UNIVERSAL PRECAUTIONS

- Gloves must be worn while performing wart, corn or callus removal
- Evaluate the need for face and eye protection.

OBTAIN INFORMED CONSENT

- Introduce yourself to the patient
- Explain the procedure to the patient, as well as the risks and benefits
- Explain expected side effects that may include pain, tenderness, erythema or blistering
- Gain informed consent to continue.

WART REMOVAL

- Warts disrupt normal skin markings and have dark specks (capillary thromboses)
- Indications
  - Medical indications are pain or tenderness
- Contraindications
  - None
- Complications
  - Hypopigmentation
  - Side effects of erythema and blistering
- Equipment
  - Scalpel
  - Liquid nitrogen
  - Alcohol swab
- Positioning
  - Make patient comfortable
- Preparation
  - Pare wart prior to procedure to better penetrate wart with liquid nitrogen
    - Clean site with alcohol prior to paring
    - Patient may attempt this at home prior to removal with nail file or pumice stone
    - Provider may pare in the office with a scalpel blade
  - Anesthesia not necessary
- Procedure
  - Cryotherapy with liquid nitrogen
    - Freeze the lesion with 2 mm of margin
    - Thaw in 30–60 seconds for common, plantar, or palmar warts
    - Thaw in 10 seconds for flat warts
    - Two freeze-thaw cycles may lead to improved resolution
  - Apply petrolatum to blister after it ruptures. Usually heals within one week.

DIFFERENTIATING CALLOSITIES

- Corns and calluses are areas of thick, hard skin, formed by friction
  - Corns usually affect the bottoms of the feet and sides of the toes, looks like a small bump, and has a hard center surrounded by an area of irritated skin. It can be painful.

- Calluses often form on the hands, fingers, feet, or toes. They look like thick, rough, sometimes bumpy skin. Calluses usually do not hurt and do not have a core.

CORN AND CALLUS REMOVAL

- Skin lines are prominent in callouses and corns instead of disrupted as with warts
- Indication
  - Discomfort, pain, change in gait
- Contraindication
  - None
- Complication
  - Irritation and tenderness are expected side effects, not complications
- Basic equipment
  - Salicylic acid plaster
  - Scissors
  - Tape
  - #15 scalpel
  - Alcohol swab
- Positioning
  - Position the patient comfortably
  - Counsel patient to ensure footwear fits properly to decrease friction
- Preparation
  - Verify that the patient does not have a peripheral neuropathy
    - May not feel pain caused by improper patch placement. Do not apply patch to neuropathic patients
  - Trim the salicylic acid plaster to the size of the lesion
- Procedure
  - Clean the lesion with alcohol swab
  - Pare through the thick skin of the corn or callus with a #15 scalpel
  - Apply plaster to lesion site, tape in place
    - Patient is to remove white skin with a metal nail file or pumice stone each night
    - Use of the patch should stop once the lesion has resolved or within 72 hours. Keep dry
  - Follow up if not resolved in 1–2 weeks

SELF-ASSESSMENT QUIZ

1. Which of the following statements are false?
   a. Corns and calluses are the same
   b. Cutaneous warts are benign proliferations of skin caused by HPV infection
   c. Corns have a central core of keratin
   d. Callouses are diffuse thickening of stratum corneum
2. What are the common locations of corns?
   a. Bottom of the feet   b. Sides of the toes
   c. Fingers   d. All of the above
   e. A and B only
3. Which skin lesion is painful?
   a. Wart   b. Corn
   c. Calluses   d. None
4. What piece of equipment is common to the removal process of each type of lesion?
   a. Liquid nitrogen   b. Salicylic acid
   c. Scalpel   d. Electrocautery
5. What features are not present in warts?
   a. Disrupted skin lines   b. Raised areas of skin
   c. Dark specks in the lesion   d. Prominent skin lines

Answers

1. a   2. e   3. b   4. c   5. d

SUGGESTED READING

1. Bae JM, Kang H, Kim HO, Park YM. Differential diagnosis of plantar wart from corn, callus and healed wart with the aid of dermoscopy. Br J Dermatol. 2009;160:220.
2. Berth-Jones J, Bourke J, Eglitis H, et al. Value of a second freeze-thaw cycle in cryotherapy of common warts. Br J Dermatol. 1994;131:883.
3. Freeman DB. Corns and calluses resulting from mechanical hyperkeratosis. Am Fam Physician. 2002;65(11):2277-80.
4. Kilkenny M, Marks R. The descriptive epidemiology of warts in the community. Austral J Dermatol. 1996;37:80.
5. Mann RA. Pain in the foot. Evaluation of foot pain and identification of associated problems. Postgrad Med. 1987;82(1):154-7.
6. Murphy GA. Lesser Toe Abnormalities: Corns (Helomata and Clavi). In: Canale ST (Ed). Campbell's Operative Orthopaedics. 10th. St. Louis, Mo: Mosby; 2003:4063-5.
7. Singh D, Bentley G, Trevino SG. Callosities, corns, and calluses. BMJ. 1996;312(7043):1403-6.
8. Snider RK. Corns and Calluses. In: Greene WB (Ed). Essentials of Musculoskeletal Care, 2nd edition. Rosemont, Ill: American Academy of Orthopaedic Surgeons; 2001. p. 437-41.

Fine Needle Aspiration

Milan S

OBJECTIVES

- Describe technique of fine needle aspiration (FNA)
- Be aware of the indications for FNA
- Describe the complications of FNA
- Be able to perform FNA

INTRODUCTION/BACKGROUND

- This minimally invasive technique involves collecting cells with a small gauge needle from palpable nodules
- The mass can be from the breast, thyroid, lymph nodes, salivary glands and subcutaneous tissue
  - Cytology is then used to confirm benign versus malignancy
  - Used for diagnostic and possibly therapeutic purposes as in with cyst aspirations.

UNIVERSAL PRECAUTIONS

- Gloves must be worn while performing fine needle aspiration
- Aspiration should be performed using sterile technique
- Evaluate the need for face and eye protection as well as a gown.

OBTAIN INFORMED CONSENT

- Introduce yourself to the patient
- Explain the procedure to the patient, as well as the risks and benefits
- Gain informed consent to continue.

INDICATIONS

- To obtain samples of palpable masses for diagnosis
- To drain cystic lesions to provide therapy
- To differentiate benign from malignant lesions.

CONTRAINDICATIONS

- No absolute contraindications
- Consider using smaller gauge needles in anticoagulated patients.

COMPLICATIONS

- Hematoma
- Bleeding
- Pain
- Infection
- Perforation of surrounding structures
- Pneumothorax—more likely in thin patients and deep lesions.

BASIC EQUIPMENT

- 22 to 27 gauge needle
- 10 mL syringe
- 5 mL syringe
- Alcohol swab
- Gauge
- Band Aid.

POSITIONING

- Goal of positioning is to provide access to the mass while keeping the patient comfortable
  - In neck masses: Lay patient supine with towel under shoulders to slightly hyperextend the neck
  - With breast masses: Patient should sit upright with upper quadrant lesions, and lay supine with lower quadrant lesions.

PREPARATION

- No local anesthesia needed
- Label specimen tube
- Prepare the 5 ml syringe by drawing air into syringe
- With the nondominant hand, fix the mass between 2 fingers
- Clean the skin over the mass with alcohol

PROCEDURE STEPS

- Advance the needle into the mass
- With the needle tip in the mass, aspirate, moving needle clockwise within the mass to obtain cells from multiple areas
- Release suction pressure and withdraw the needle
- Remove the needle from the syringe, attach needle to empty syringe and expel specimen from needle into container.

SPECIMEN ANALYSIS

- Send biopsy specimen for analysis
- If fluid aspirated, may also be sent for analysis

SELF-ASSESSMENT QUIZ

1. What kind of mass is fine needle aspiration not used on?
   - a. Breast
   - b. Lymph node
   - c. Ovarian
   - d. Salivary gland
2. What is a fine needle aspiration used for?
   - a. To obtain samples of palpable masses for diagnosis
   - b. To drain cystic lesions to provide therapy
   - c. To differentiate benign from malignant lesions
   - d. All of the above
3. What option is not a part of the preparation prior to aspiration?
   - a. Prepare the 5 mL syringe by drawing air into syringe
   - b. Administer local anesthesia
   - c. With the nondominant hand, fix the mass between 2 fingers
   - d. Clean the skin over the mass with alcohol
4. What potential complication could be immediately life-threatening?
   - a. Pneumothorax
   - b. Pain
   - c. Bleeding
   - d. Infection
5. What is the best position for an aspiration?
   - a. Neck mass: Head in neutral position
   - b. Breast mass: Sit up with lower quadrant masses
   - c. Breast mass: Lay supine with lower quadrant masses
   - d. Breast mass: Lay supine with upper quadrant lesions

Answers

1. c   2. d   3. b   4. a   5. c

SUGGESTED READING

1. Amedee RG, Dhurandhar NR. Fine-needle aspiration biopsy. Laryngoscope. 2001;111(9):1551-7.
2. Britton PD. Fine needle aspiration or core biopsy. Breast. 1999;8(1):1-4.
3. DeMay RM. Practical Principles of Cytopathology. Chicago: American Society for Cytopathology; 2007.
4. Liu K, Dodge R, Glasgow BJ, Layfield LJ. Fine-needle aspiration: comparison of smear, cytospin, and cell block preparations in diagnostic and cost effectiveness. Diagn Cytopathol. 1998;19(1):70-4.
5. Nasuti JF, Gupta PK, Baloch ZW. Diagnostic value and cost-effectiveness of on-site evaluation of fine-needle aspiration specimens: review of 5,688 cases. Diagn Cytopathol. 2002;27(1):1-4.
6. Orell SR, Sterrett GF, Walters MN, Whitaker D. The techniques of FNA cytology. In: Manual and Atlas of Fine Needle Aspiration Cytology. 3rd ed. London, England: Churchill Livingstone; 1999. p. 12-13.
7. Rubin E, Farber JL. Pathology, 2nd ed. Philadelphia, PA: Lippincott Williams & Wilkins, 1994.
8. Shah KA. Fine needle aspiration. J Laryngol Otol. 2003;117(6):493-5.
9. Stanley MW, Lowhagen T. Basic Techniques. In: Fine Needle Aspiration of Palpable Masses. Boston, MA: Butterworth-Heinemann; 1993. p. 18-56.

Breast Cyst Aspiration

Milan S

INTRODUCTION/BACKGROUND

• Aspiration may be attempted in cases of a palpable, dominant breast mass
• If clear fluid is aspirated and the mass resolves a breast cyst is the most likely diagnosis. Reevaluate in 4–6 weeks for recurrence
• If the aspirate is bloody, mass did not resolve, or no fluid was aspirated, fine needle or excisional biopsy is indicated.

UNIVERSAL PRECAUTIONS

• Gloves must be worn while performing aspiration
• Evaluate the need for face and eye protection as well as a gown.

OBTAIN INFORMED CONSENT

• Introduce yourself to the patient
• Explain the procedure to the patient, as well as the risks and benefit
• Gain informed consent to continue.

INDICATIONS

• Evaluation of palpable breast mass
  – To determine benign vs malignant
• Aspiration of breast cysts.

CONTRAINDICATIONS

- Multiple masses
- Lack of dominant mass.

COMPLICATIONS

- Bleeding
- Hematoma
- Infection
- Pain at aspiration site
- Pneumothorax.

BASIC EQUIPMENT

- Skin prep solution
- Gloves
- 21–22 gauge needle
- 5 mL syringe
- Bandage.

SITES/POSITIONING

- For upper quadrant lesions
  - Place the patient in a seated upright position
- For lower quadrant lesions
  - Place the patient supine.

PREPARATION

- Clean skin overlying mass with skin prep (povidone-iodine solution, followed by alcohol swab)
- Place sterile drapes around the site to reduce the risk of infection
- Put on sterile gloves
- Attach needle to syringe.

PROCEDURE STEPS

- Locate the mass and fix the mass between index and middle finger of the nondominant hand
- Insert needle, aiming at the center of the mass
- Apply suction pressure to aspirate cyst contents
  - If no fluid is aspirated, adjust the needle placement to ensure the cyst was punctured
- Release aspiration pressure, withdraw needle
- Apply bandage to aspiration site.

SELF-ASSESSMENT QUIZ

1. Breast cysts are usually formed because of:
    a. Duct obstruction
    b. Involution changes
    c. Aging of ducts
    d. All of the above
    e. None of the above
2. Breast cysts are a common cause of palpable breast masses in:
    a. Adolescent patients
    b. Patients between 20 and 39 years
    c. Patients between 40 and 50 years
    d. Postmenopausal patients not receiving hormonal therapy
3. A 41-year-old patient presents to a rural health clinic with a palpable right breast mass measuring 2 x 1.7 cm. The lesion is well delineated and mobile, with smooth margins. Regional lymph nodes are not enlarged, and there are no skin changes, nipple retraction and discharge. Six months ago the patient had normal screening mammogram. What it the best next step at this time?
    a. Perform breast cyst aspiration
    b. Repeat mammography
    c. Perform MRI of the breast
    d. None of the above
4. Choose the most appropriate sequence of the steps for breast cyst aspiration:
    a. Place sterile drapes around the aspiration site, clean skin with skin prep, insert needle at the periphery of the mass and aspirate the content
    b. Clean skin overlying mass with skin prep, place sterile drapes around the aspiration site, locate breast mass, insert needle aiming the center of the mass and apply suction pressure to aspirate the content
    c. Clean skin with skin prep, locate breast mass, insert needle to the center of the mass and apply pressure to aspirate the content
    d. Drape the patient, clean skin area, insert the needle to the bottom of the breast lesion and aspirate the content
5. Follow-up of the patient following breast cyst aspiration includes:
    a. Assessment of the aspirate
    b. Palpation of the cyst after aspiration to assure complete resolution
    c. Revaluation of the patient 4–6 weeks
    d. Referral of the patient for surgical biopsy if the cyst is being refilled or there is a residual mass
    e. All of the above
    f. None of the above

Answers

1. d   2. c   3. a   4. b   5. e

SUGGESTED READING

1. Cady B, Steele GD Jr, Morrow M, Gardner B, Smith BL, Lee NC, et al. Evaluation of common breast problems: Guidance for primary care providers. CA Cancer J Clin. 1998;48:49-63.

2. Delva D, Tomalty L, Payne P. Fine needle aspiration of breast lumps. Can Fam Physician. 2002;48:1055-6.

3. Henson RM, Wyatt SW, Lee NC. The National Breast and Cervical Cancer Early Detection Program: a comprehensive public health response to two major health issues for women. J Public Health Manag Pract. 1996;2:36-47.

4. Hindle WH, Arias RD, Florentine B, Whang J. Lack of utility in clinical practice of cytologic examination of nonbloody cyst fluid from palpable breast cysts. Am J Obstet Gynecol. 2000;182:1300-5.

5. Lamm RL, Jackman RJ. Mammographic abnormalities caused by percutaneous stereotactic biopsy of histologically benign lesions evident on follow-up mammograms. Am J Roentgenol. 2001;174:753-6.

6. Lucas J, Cone L. Breast Cyst Aspiration. American Family Physician. 2003;68(10):1983-6.

7. Morrow M. The evaluation of common breast problems. Am Fam Physician. 2000;61:2371-8.,2385.

Skin Biopsies: Punch, Shave and Excisional

Milan S

INTRODUCTION/BACKGROUND

- Skin biopsies are often performed when patients present with a dermatologic lesion that cannot be clinically identified
- Biopsies can be performed in office with tissue sent to pathology
  - Punch, shave and excisional biopsies have differing indications for their use
  - Select the appropriate therapy by the lesion appearance and type.

UNIVERSAL PRECAUTIONS

- Gloves must be worn while preparing for biopsies
- Biopsy procedures should be performed using sterile technique
- Evaluate the need for face and eye protection as well as a gown.

OBTAIN INFORMED CONSENT

- Introduce yourself to the patient
- Explain the procedure to the patient, as well as the risks and benefits
- Gain informed consent to continue.

PUNCH BIOPSY

- Indications
  - Obtains diagnostic full-thickness skin specimens for:

- Superficial inflammatory diseases
- Papulosquamous disorders
- Connective tissue disorders
- Superficial bullous diseases
- Benign tumors
- Granulomatous diseases
- Nonmelanotic malignant tumors

- Contraindications
  - Skin biopsy is rarely contraindicated
  - Routine biopsy of skin rashes is not recommended because the commonly reported nonspecific pathology result rarely alters clinical management
- Complications
  - Bleeding
  - Hematoma
  - Infection
  - Failure to heal
- Basic equipment
  - Gloves, iodine, specimen container
  - Gauze, antibiotic ointment, bandaid
  - Iris scissors
  - Sterile fenestrated drape, sterile gloves
  - 3 mL syringe, 2% lidocaine with epinephrine, 30 gauge needle
  - Punch biopsy instrument (3 or 4 mm)
  - Needle holder, suture (4-0 to 6-0 nylon)
- Site
  - The area to be biopsied should be selected
  - Commonly selected sites are the most abnormal-appearing site within a lesion or the edge of an actively growing lesion
  - Identify the lines of least skin tension
    - The suture placed after biopsy should allow the skin to close parallel to the line of least tension
- Preparation
  - Clean area with iodine and anesthetize with 2% lidocaine with epinephrine
  - Put on sterile gloves and drape area
  - Stretch the skin around the biopsy site with the thumb and index finger perpendicular to the line of least tension
    - When the skin relaxes after the biopsy an elliptical-shaped wound remains in the same direction as the lines of least skin tension
- Procedure steps
  - Hold the instrument vertically over the skin
  - Rotate downward with a twisting motion

- Once the instrument is in the subcutaneous fat or to the hub, remove the instrument
- Elevate the specimen with the tip of the needle and cut the specimen free with scissors below the dermis
- Achieve hemostasis of the wound
  - For simple oozing, the suture will be enough to achieve hemostasis
- Close the wound with 1–2 interrupted simple sutures
  - 6-0 nylon on the face
  - 5-0 nylon most all other locations
- Apply antibiotic ointment and bandage.

SHAVE BIOPSY

- Indications
  - Removal of raised lesion, lesion that easily separates from skin, dome-shaped nevi, benign tumors, nonmelanotic malignant tumors
- Contraindications
  - Lesion concerning for melanoma
- Complications
  - Infection, bleeding, scarring, failure to heal
- Basic equipment
  - No. 15 scalpel or bowed metal razor blade
  - 2% Lidocaine with epinephrine
  - 25 gauge needle, 3–5 cc syringe
  - Cleaning solution, forceps, gauze, Band Aid
- Preparation
  - Clean site with betadine or alcohol
  - Inject anesthetic around base and under lesion
- Procedure
  - Stretch and stabilize skin with nondominant hand
    - If the lesion is flat, pinch upward with forceps
  - Hold the blade horizontal to the skin
  - Begin the cut just outside the lesion's border
  - Cut with a single smooth cutting stroke
  - Achieve hemostasis after procedure.

EXCISIONAL BIOPSY

- Indications
  - Provides both diagnosis and therapy
- Also known as elliptical excision of:
  - Subcutaneous lesions
  - Deep dermal tumors

- Deep inflammatory diseases (erythema nodosum)
- Malignant melanoma
- Any atypical pigmented lesions suspicious for melanoma
- Contraindications
  - Skin biopsy is rarely contraindicated
  - Bleeding disorders or anticoagulated patients may have prolonged bleeding but this is not a contraindication
- Complications
  - Bleeding at the site
  - Hematoma formation
  - Infection
- Basic equipment
  - Nonsterile
    - Gloves, skin marking pen, cleaning solution
    - Gauze, syringe with 2% lidocaine with epinephrine, 25 gauge needle, electrocautery
  - Sterile
    - Sterile gloves, fenestrated drape
    - Scissors, forceps, 4 × 4 gauze
    - Skin hook or 21 gauge needle to be bent into skin hooks
    - Needle holder, 4-0, 5-0 or 6-0 nylon sutures
- Biopsy site
  - The size of the excision depends upon lesion diameter and appropriate margin
    - 2 mm in benign excisions
    - 4 mm margin in most basal cell carcinomas
    - Melanoma in situ is a 5 mm margin for cure
  - Fusiform excisional biopsies generally extend just beyond the lesion's border
    - If the pathology report indicates the need for larger margins, re-excision can be performed
- Preparation
  - Mark the area to be biopsied
    - 3:1 length to width ratio
    - Long axis of wound parallel with lines of least skin tension
  - Anesthetize the area under the planned biopsy site
  - Clean the area with iodine, apply sterile gloves and drape the area
- Procedure steps
  - Holding the tip of the scalpel perpendicular, incise the skin at one corner of the site
  - Then lower the blade handle to use the curved edge of the blade and make a continuous incision along one side of the lesion
    - Repeat on the opposite side

- Grasp the corner of the biopsy edge with forceps and remove all layers down to the fat
- Place specimen in specimen container
- Grasp the lateral skin edges with skin hooks and undermine 3 cm for each 1 cm the skin needs to displace
    - Control bleeding beneath the skin edges with direct pressure or electrocautery
- Deep subcuticular sutures may be needed
    - Close deep space (4-0 or 5-0 polyglactin)
- Evert skin edges and close wound with interrupted simple nylon sutures.

INCISIONAL BIOPSY

- Incisional (also known as wedge) biopsy can be performed on lesions that cannot be completely excised
- Uses fusiform excision technique, however the borders will be within the lesion
    - Biopsy site should be either central, dark or suspicious-looking areas and large enough to have adequate tissue for pathology.

POST-PROCEDURE CONCERNS

- Pathology submission:
    - Handle biopsy specimens carefully to minimize crush injury
    - Label each with the biopsy site, patient name, identification number and date
    - Provide a brief summary of the patient's clinical history when you submit a biopsy specimen to assist the pathologist in creating an appropriate differential diagnosis
- Hemostasis:
    - Hemostasis can be achieved with topical application of aluminum chloride or ferric subsulfate (Monsel's) solution
    - Aluminum chloride can slow wound healing, but is preferred on facial wounds as Monsel's solution may rarely cause discolorations.

SUTURE REMOVAL

- Remove the skin sutures as early as possible, replacing them with skin tape.
    - Facial cutaneous sutures may be removed after 5–7 days
    - Truncal and extremity sutures may be removed after 10–14 days
- Failure to remove in a good timeframe can cause reepithelialization over the sutures, as well as track marks along the external path of the sutures.

SELF-ASSESSMENT QUIZ

1. When is a shave biopsy not indicated?
    a. Raised lesion   b. Dome-shaped nevi
    c. Malignant melanoma   d. Benign tumors
2. What proportion of length to width should be used in fusiform excisions?
    a. 1:2   b. 2:1
    c. 1:3   d. 3:1
3. What solutions can be used to achieve hemostasis?
    a. Monsel's solution   b. Aluminum chloride
    c. Both   d. Neither
4. What suture size should be used on the face?
    a. 6-0   b. 4-0
    c. 3-0   d. 2-0
5. What is the least preferred biopsy method for suspected malignant melanoma?
    a. Incisional biopsy   b. Shave biopsy
    c. Punch biopsy   d. Fusiform biopsy

Answers

1. c   2. d   3. c   4. a   5. b

SUGGESTED READING

1. Brown JS. Minor surgery: Text and Atlas. 3d ed. New York: Chapman & Hall; 1997.
2. Fewkes JL, Sober AJ. Skin biopsy: The four types and how best to do them. Prim Care Cancer. 1993;13:36-9.
3. Pariser RJ. Skin biopsy: Lesion selection and optimal technique. Mod Med. 1989;57:82-90.
4. Paver RD. Practical procedures in dermatology. Austr Fam Physician. 1990;19:699-701.
5. Phillips PK, Pariser DM, Pariser RJ. Cosmetic procedures we all perform. Cutis. 1994;53:187-91.
6. Pories WJ, Thomas FT, eds. Office Surgery for Family Physicians. Boston: Butterworth & Co. 1985. p. 57-64.
7. Stegman SJ. Basics of dermatologic surgery. Chicago: Year Book Medical; 1982.
8. Swanson NA. Atlas of cutaneous surgery. Boston: Little, Brown, 1987.
9. Zuber TJ, DeWitt DE. The fusiform excision. Am Fam Physician. 1994;49:371-6.
10. Zuber TJ. Skin biopsy techniques: When and how to perform punch biopsy. Consultant. 1994;34:1467-70.

Incision and Drainage of Superficial Skin Abscesses

Milan S

OBJECTIVES

- Describe incision and drainage technique of superficial skin abscess
- List the indications for incision and drainage (I & D) of superficial skin abscess
- Describe the complications of I & D of superficial skin abscess
- Know how to perform I & D of skin abscess

INTRODUCTION/BACKGROUND

- Skin abscesses are collections of pus in and below the dermis and should be incised and drained
  - Are not infections of the hair follicles
- Most abscesses are polymicrobial, with aerobic as well as anaerobic bacteria
  - *Staphylococcus aureus* is a facultative anaerobe, able to reproduce in both aerobic and anaerobic conditions.

UNIVERSAL PRECAUTIONS

- Sterile gloves must be worn while performing incision and drainage
- Eye protection should be worn
- Evaluate the need for face protection as well as a gown.

OBTAIN INFORMED CONSENT

- Introduce yourself to the patient
- Explain the procedure to the patient, as well as the risks and benefits
- Gain informed consent and explain
  - Abscess may be larger than it appears
  - Scar can form at incision site
  - Recurrence may occur.

INDICATIONS

- All except small abscesses that spontaneously drain should be incised and drained
- A small draining abscess could be observed, with warm compresses applied to encourage continued drainage
- Needle aspiration has been shown to not provide a large enough tract to adequately drain the skin abscesses.

CONTRAINDICATIONS

- Perirectal abscesses have a high rate of fistula formation and if recurrent should follow up with a surgeon
- Neck, breast, hand and abscesses located near complicated anatomy may need precise drainage by a surgeon
- Facial abscesses should be treated with antibiotics and referred to otolaryngology
- Coagulopathies should be corrected.

COMPLICATIONS

- Lack of proper drainage can lead to local extension
  - Osteomyelitis, tenosynovitis, septic thrombophlebitis, necrotizing fasciitis, or fistula formation
- Dissection may damage nearby structures
- Bacteremia
- Secondary infections.

BASIC EQUIPMENT

- Sterile skin preparation solution
- Sterile gloves, 4 × 4 gauze and drapes
- Scalpel, basin, sterile saline, 30 mL syringe
- Curved hemostats, forceps, scissors
- 10 mL syringe, 25 gauge needle, lidocaine
- Culture swab
- Packing gauze
- Sterile 2 × 2 gauze and tape.

SITES/POSITIONING

- Position patient for comfort and accessibility of abscess site
- Sterile prep and drape the site.

PREPARATION

- Local anesthesia can be ineffective due to the altered pH
  - Field block may be required: Application of anesthetic around the entire wound circumference
- Insert needle into abscess to obtain sterile sample for microbiology
- Packing placement
  - >5 cm in diameter, in immunocompromised or diabetic patient, or pilonidal abscess.

PROCEDURE STEPS

- Incise the skin with a linear incision over the area of greatest fluctuance
- If the abscess is in a cosmetic area or an area of skin tension, a stab incision may be used to limit tissue injury and scarring
- Break up loculations with hemostat
- Irrigate the abscess cavity with saline until all visible pus is removed, then pack the wound
- Tape absorbent dressing over wound.

ASPIRATE ANALYSIS

- Send Gram stain, culture and sensitivity testing if the patient will be treated with antibiotics or if the patient has
  - Severe local infection
  - Systemic infection
  - Recurrent or multiple abscesses
  - Failure of antibiotic treatment
  - Very young or old patient
  - Immunocompromised patients.

FOLLOW-UP

- Advise patient to seek care in case of
  - Fever or chills, increased pain, edema, erythema or reaccumulation of pus
- The primary care physician should re-examine the wound within 24 to 48 hours.
  - If needed, the wound may be debrided or enlarged
  - Packing should be changed.

SELF-ASSESSMENT QUIZ

1. What can be a complication of not correctly draining an abscess?
    a. Osteomyelitis
    b. Tenosynovitis
    c. Fistula formation
    d. All of the above
2. For which patient should the aspirate be sent for testing?
    a. Healthy adult
    b. Teenager with their first cyst
    c. Adult with sepsis
    d. Adult on their first antibiotic
3. Which of the following is a complication of an I & D?
    a. Damage of nearby structures
    b. Bacteremia
    c. Secondary infections
    d. All of the above
4. Which sized cyst will need wound packing after drainage?
    a. 0.5 cm in diameter
    b. 2 cm in diameter
    c. 4 cm in diameter
    d. 6 cm in diameter
5. When should the patient follow-up early?
    a. Fever or chills
    b. Controlled pain
    c. Minimal local erythema
    d. Decreasing amount of pus

Answers

1. d   2. c   3. d   4. d   5. a

SUGGESTED READING

1. Butler K. Incision and Drainage. Clinical Procedures in Emergency Medicine, 5th ed. Philadelphia, PA: Saunder Elsevier. 2010. p. 657.
2. Daly, L, Durani, Y. Incision and drainage of a cutaneous abscess. Textbook of Pediatric Emergency Procedures, 2nd ed. Philadelphia, PA: Mosby, Elsevier; 2008. p. 1079.
3. Derkson, DJ. Incision and drainage of an abscess. In: Pfenninger, J, Fowler, GC (Eds). Procedures for primary care physicians, 1st ed. St Luis: Mosby; 1994. p. 50.
4. Fitch MT, Manthey DE, McGinnis HD, et al. Videos in clinical medicine. Abscess incision and drainage. N Engl J Med. 2007;357:e20.
5. Halvorson GD, Halvorson JE, Iserson KV. Abscess incision and drainage in the emergency department. J Emerg Med. 1985;3:227.
6. Korownyk C, Allan GM. Evidence-based approach to abscess management. Can Fam Physician. 2007;53:1680.
7. Singer AJ, Taira BR, Chale S, et al. Primary versus secondary closure of cutaneous abscesses in the emergency department: A randomized controlled trial. Acad Emerg Med. 2013;20:27.
8. Singer AJ, Thode HC Jr, Chale S, et al. Primary closure of cutaneous abscesses: A systematic review. Am J Emerg Med. 2011;29:361.

Removal of Foreign Bodies, Rings and Fishhooks

Newbrough B

OBJECTIVES

- Describe removal technique for rings, foreign bodies and fishhooks
- List the indications for specialist referral
- Be able to determine the specific technique to use based on the situation
- Describe the complications of the removal of foreign bodies
- Know how to perform removal of foreign bodies, rings and fishhooks

INTRODUCTION/BACKGROUND

- Foreign bodies in the ear and nose are removed by different techniques
  - Including forceps, water irrigation or suction
- Removal of rings prevent vascular compromise with multiple methods
  - Band cutting, string wrap, elastic pull
- Fishhook injuries are typically minor but removal has multiple techniques as well
  - Retrograde, advance and cut, string-yank.

UNIVERSAL PRECAUTIONS

- Gloves must be worn while performing these procedures
- Evaluate the need for face and eye protection
  - May be needed with fishhook or ring removal to prevent provider injuries.

OBTAIN INFORMED CONSENT

- Introduce yourself to the patient
- Explain the procedure to the patient, as well as the risks and benefits
- Gain informed consent to continue.

FOREIGN BODY REMOVAL

- Indications
  - Foreign bodies in ear or nose
- Contraindications
  - If trauma to the area, object cannot be properly visualized or attempts are unsuccessful, refer to ENT or HNS
- Complications
  - Bleeding, trauma
  - Ear: Decreased hearing
  - Nasal: May descend into the oropharynx
- Ear foreign body removal
  - Basic equipment
    - Forceps, cerumen loop, suction catheter or right angle ball hook
    - Otoscope with removable lens
    - Headlamp
    - Syringe and 20 gauge angiocatheter
    - Acetone, 2% lidocaine, mineral oil, alcohol in specific circumstances
  - Preparation
    - Position patient by provider's preference
      - Seated
      - Lateral decubitus
    - Gently retract the pinna superiorly and posteriorly to straighten the ear canal for optimal visualization
  - Techniques
    - Syringe and angiocath irrigation with water–not if object is a battery
    - Grasping with forceps, cerumen loop, suction catheter, or right angle ball hook
    - Acetone to dissolve styrofoam or loosen superglue
    - Live insects can be killed with alcohol, 2% lidocaine or mineral oil if tympanic membrane is not ruptured
- Nasal foreign body removal
  - Basic equipment
    - Light source
    - 0.5% phenylephrine, topical lidocaine
    - Nasal speculum
    - Bag-valve mask
    - Forceps, hooked probe, curette
    - Balloon catheter
    - Suction apparatus
  - Preparation
    - Position patient in the sniffing position
      - Supine or with slight elevation of the head
      - Uncooperative patients must be securely immobilized

- 0.5% phenylephrine to reduce mucosal edema, topical lidocaine for analgesia
  - Techniques
    - Grasp with forceps, cerumen loop, suction catheter, or curved hook
    - Blow nose or positive pressure ventilation to mouth
      - With other nostril obstructed
    - Lubricated balloon tip catheter for posterior objects
      - Pass uninflated beyond the object, inflate then pull forward, moving object anteriorly
    - 0.5% phenylephrine to reduce mucosal edema, topical lidocaine for analgesia.

RING REMOVAL

- Indications
  - Remove rapidly if absent capillary refill, gray or mottled color (vascular compromise)
  - Remove prior to swelling in extremity trauma
- Contraindications
  - No absolute contraindications
- Complications
  - Soft tissue trauma, bruising, laceration
- Basic equipment
  - Lidocaine, 25 G needle, 5 cc syringe
  - Iodine, betadine or chlorhexidine
  - Penrose drain, suture line, or elastic band
  - Soap and water or lubricant
  - Ring cutters
- Preparation
  - Make sure patient is comfortable
    - Local anesthetic or digital block
  - Clean with iodine prior to removal
  - Consider need for tetanus toxoid
  - Reduce swelling: Apply ice and elevate
    - Can also wrap Penrose drain under ring
  - Lubricate the ring
    - Apply soap or water-soluble lubricant liberally
- Procedure steps
  - Ring cutting
    - Perform if neurovascular compromise or if open wound, fracture, or dislocation distal to the ring
    - Place the guard of the ring cutter under the ring on palmar or plantar surface

- Turn the saw blade wheel on the ring, making sure it does not get too hot
- Place gauze under the cut edge and make a second cut to remove the ring
  - Elastic pull method
    - Use 2.0 or 3.0 silk, or elastic band (Penrose drain, oxygen mask strap, rubber band, phlebotomy tourniquet)
    - Grasp the band and pull with some rotation around the axis
    - Moving the band to different areas on the ring to work it further down the digit
    - Ring will gradually move positions and come off
  - String wrap method
    - Loop one end of 2.0/3.0 suture or Penrose drain under the ring
    - With the free end, wrap tightly around the digit and overlap wraps, continue wrapping beyond the proximal interphalangeal joint
    - Once the wrapping is complete, pull on the proximal end of the wrapping material so that the ring is removed.

FISHHOOK REMOVAL

- Indications
  - All embedded fishhooks should be removed
  - Prevent infection and minimize tissue trauma
  - Also consider need for tetanus toxoid
- Contraindications
  - None, however, fishhooks in the orbital region should be sent to ophthalmology
- Complications
  - Tissue trauma, infection, poor healing
- Basic equipment
  - Forceps
  - Clamp
  - 25 G needle, 10 mL syringe
  - Iodine, alcohol, or chlorhexidine
  - Wire cutters
- Preparations
  - Take note of type, size, barb presence
    - Hooks with multiple barbs should have nonembedded barbs taped to prevent injury
  - Make sure patient is comfortable
    - Pain control: Local anesthetic or digital/nerve block
  - Clean area with povidone-iodine or hexachlorophene prior to attempting removal

- Procedure steps
  - Removal techniques with least amount of trauma
    - Retrograde: Good for barbless and superficial hooks. Downward pressure on the hook helps disengage the barb from tissue, then back up along entry path
    - String-yank method: Good for deeply embedded hooks, requires fixed body part. String is wrapped around fishhook at mid-bend. Stabilize skin and put pressure on eye of fishhook. Yank string along angle of entry
  - Advance and cut method: Very successful, even with large hooks. Advance fishhook until hook point penetrates skin
    - Single point hooks
      - Cut barbed point off then back hook out through original entry site
    - Multiple barbs
      - Cut fishhook eye off and continue to advance hook forward.

SELF-ASSESSMENT QUIZ

1. What removal technique is an option for a nasal foreign body that is not an option for the ear?
   a. Grasping with forceps
   b. Grasping with cerumen loop
   c. Suction by catheter
   d. Positive pressure
2. How do you remove a nasal foreign body that positioned posteriorly?
   a. Irrigation with water
   b. Lubricated balloon tip catheter
   c. Multiple grasping attempts With forceps
   d. Pushing the object further posterior with forceps
3. What ring removal method should be used on a patient with vascular compromise of the digit?
   a. Ring cutting method
   b. Elastic pull method
   c. String wrap method
   d. String yank method
4. Which method of fishhook removal creates the most tissue trauma?
   a. Retrograde
   b. String yank
   c. Advance and cut
   d. None
5. What is an option to remove a styrofoam foreign body from the ear that would not be used for any other foreign body?
   a. Irrigation with water
   b. Grasping with a suction catheter
   c. Acetone
   d. 2% lidocaine

Answers

1. d   2. b   3. a   4. c   5. c

SUGGESTED READING

1. Backlin Sa. Positive-pressure technique for nasal foreign body removal in children. Ann Emerg Med. 1995;25:554-5.
2. Baker A, et al. The occasional ring removal. Can J Rural Med. 2010;15:26.
3. Chan Tc, Et Al. Nasal foreign body removal. J Emerg Med. 2004;26:441-5.
4. Chiu Tf, et al. Use of a penrose drain to remove an entrapped ring from a finger under emergent conditions. Am J Emerg Med. 2007;25:722.
5. Cresap Cr. Removal of a hardened steel ring from an extremely swollen finger. Am J Emerg Med. 1995;13:318.
6. Dimuzio J Jr, Deschler Dg. Emergency department management of foreign bodies of the external ear canal in children. Otol Neurotol. 2002;23:473-5.
7. Fox Jr. Fogarty catheter removal of nasal foreign bodies. Ann Emerg Med. 1980;9:37.
8. Kalan A, Tariq M. Foreign bodies in the nasal cavities: A comprehensive review of the aetiology, diagnostic pointers, and therapeutic measures. Postgrad Med J. 2000;76:484-7.
9. Lantsberg L, Blintsovsky E, Hoda J. How to extract an indwelling fishhook. Am Fam Physician. 1992;45:2589-90.
10. White Sj, Broner S. The use of Acetone to dissolve a styrofoam impaction of the Ear. Ann Emerg Med. 1994;23:580-2.

Control of Epistaxis

Newbrough B, Milan S

OBJECTIVES

- Describe the correct escalation of techniques for control of epistaxis
- List the indications for packing and cautery for control of epistaxis
- Describe the complications of packing and cautery
- Know how to perform techniques for control of epistaxis in the proper order indicated

INTRODUCTION/BACKGROUND

- Causes include trauma, coagulation disorders, platelet dysfunction, vascular lesions, nasal tumors and hereditary telangiectasia
    - Hypertension does not cause epistaxis but may prolong the bleeding
- Stop bleeding by starting at the most basic intervention
- Increase levels only if needed.

UNIVERSAL PRECAUTIONS

- Gloves must be worn
- Evaluate the need for face and eye protection as well as a gown, as a patient with epistaxis who sneezes can produce a spray of blood.

OBTAIN INFORMED CONSENT

- Introduce yourself to the patient
- Explain the procedure to the patient, as well as the risks and benefits
- Patients need to be made aware of signs, symptoms and risks of toxic shock syndrome with any form of nasal packing. Risks increase with retention of packing materials greater than 72 hours
- Gain informed consent to continue.

INDICATIONS

- Recurrent episodes of epistaxis
- Suspected epistaxis as visualized by hematemesis or melena
    - Potential presentation of posterior epistaxis
- Direct pressure failed to stop the bleeding.

CONTRAINDICATIONS

- No absolute contraindications
- Patients with respiratory compromise may need airway support prior to focusing on the epistaxis
- Patients that may need to go to the emergency department
    - Known coagulopathic patient
    - Known platelet dysfunction
    - Hemodynamic compromise.

COMPLICATIONS

- Intranasal adhesions
- Aspiration
- Hypoxic complications
- Treatment failure or dislodgment
- Septal necrosis
- Toxic shock syndrome
- Sinus or nasolacrimal infections.

BASIC EQUIPMENT

- 2% lidocaine with epinephrine
- Oxymetazoline, phenylephrine or epinephrine
- Gloves, eye shield, gown
- Headlamp, nasal speculum
- Tape, cotton, tongue depressors
- Silver nitrate, nasal tampon, Rapid Rhino™, Merocel nasal packing.

SITE OF BLEEDING

- Examine both nares with a nasal speculum
    - If source seen: Cauterize with silver nitrate or electrocautery. If bleeding continues after cautery, perform nasal packing
    - If no bleeding is identified, the patient should be taught basic tamponade technique and instructed to return in case of recurrence.

PREPARATION

- Topical anesthetic
  - 2% lidocaine with epinephrine
- Topical vasoconstrictor
  - Oxymetazoline, phenylephrine, epinephrine
- Position patient upright, not reclined.

PROCEDURE STEPS

- Conservative measures
- Cautery if discrete bleed visualized
- Anterior nasal packing
  - Nasal tampon, balloon catheter or gauze
  - Any packing to be removed at 48–72 hours
- Bilateral packing
- Posterior packing
- ENT or surgery referral.

CONSERVATIVE MEASURES

- Two sprays of oxymetazoline in each nostril
- Pinch alae tightly against the septum and hold continuously for 15 minutes
- Patient to bend forward at waist with a cotton wool plug inside the nose and a cold compress on the bridge of the nose.

CHEMICAL CAUTERY

- Silver nitrate
  - Apply the applicator tip proximally at the periphery of the bleeding site and move towards the center for a maximum of 10 seconds
  - Will not work if area is too bloody, suction may be used to dry area
  - Remove excess silver nitrate with cotton
  - Do not cauterize both nares (can cause septal necrosis).

ANTERIOR NASAL PACKING

- Nasal tampon
  - Coat with bacitracin ointment and slide along the floor of the nasal cavity, leaving the tip exposed
  - Expand it with 10 mL of saline
- Gauze packing
  - With forceps, stack layers of ribbon gauze onto the floor of the nasal cavity, folding gauze into place

- Nasal balloon catheter
  - Soak Rapid Rhino™ in sterile water for 30 seconds (becomes slick)
  - Insert along the floor of the nasal cavity until the plastic ring lies inside the nare
  - Inflate balloon with air using 20 cc syringe, stop when pilot cuff is firm
  - Ensure cuff still firm in 15 minutes, reinflate if needed
  - Tape cuff to patient's cheek.

BILATERAL PACKING

- If bleeding continues in spite of packing
  - Contralateral naris may be packed, which acts as a counterforce
- If bilateral anterior packing fails to produce hemostasis, the patient likely has a posterior bleed
  - Treat for a posterior bleed
  - Consider need for hospitalization with a cardiac monitor for any posterior bleed, or for those unlikely to follow up.

POSTERIOR PACKING

- Double nasal balloon catheter
  - Has an anterior and a posterior balloon
  - Advance the catheter along the floor of the nasal cavity until the retention ring reaches the naris and inflate the posterior balloon
  - Retract the catheter gently until it lodges posteriorly, then inflate the anterior balloon
  - Pad and protect the alae and naris entrance
- If no nasal balloon, use a Foley catheter
  - Coat with a petroleum-free lubricant, trim the tip of the catheter and advance along the floor until visualized in the oropharynx
  - Inject 5 mL of sterile saline in the balloon and retract until it lodges against the posterior choana and add 5 mL more
  - Clamp the catheter in place with an umbilical clamp. Pad to prevent excessive pressure
  - Anterior pack may be performed per clinician preference
- Posterior cotton pack
  - Insert a small caliber red rubber tube through the nose and draw it out the oropharynx with forceps
  - Tie a cotton pack to the tube's oral end and retract the hose until it lodges against the posterior choana
  - With the ties, secure a second cotton pack or gauze roll into the nasal end
  - Also apply an anterior packing.

SPECIALIST REFERRAL

- Immediate otolaryngologic (ENT) consultation is necessary if bleeding is heavy and cannot be controlled with posterior packing
- If packing was placed, the patient should follow-up with ENT at 24–48 hours
    - ENT will likely remove packing to inspect the site and determine need for further intervention.

SELF-ASSESSMENT QUIZ

1. Which of the following is the correct order of escalation of attempts to stop a nosebleed?

    1. Posterior nasal packing   2. Anterior nasal packing   3. ENT referral

    a. 1, 2, 3   b. 2, 3, 1
    c. 2, 1, 3   d. 3, 1, 2

2. When should nasal packing be removed?
    a. When the patient no longer tastes blood
    b. At 20 minutes
    c. At 2 hours
    d. At 2 days

3. What should you do if silver nitrate cautery does not stop the bleeding?
    a. Cauterize the other side
    b. Dry the area and retry for 10 seconds
    c. Reapply, leaving in place for 1 minute
    d. Rinse the area with saline

4. How does bilateral packing help to decrease nasal bleeding?
    a. Places pressure from both sides
    b. Allows the blood to run posteriorly
    c. Only works with an interrupted nasal septum
    d. Increased absorption

5. What specialist should see a patient that required posterior nasal packing?
    a. Hematologist   b. Oncologist
    c. Allergist   d. Otolaryngologist

Answers

1. c   2. d   3. b   4. a   5. d

SUGGESTED READING

1. Alvi A, Joyner-Triplett N. Acute epistaxis. How to spot the source and stop the flow. Postgrad Med. 1996;99:83.
2. Kotecha B, Fowler S, Harkness P, et al. Management of epistaxis: a national survey. Ann R Coll Surg Engl. 1996;78:444.
3. Kucik CJ, Clenney T. Management of epistaxis. Am Fam Physician. 2005;71:305.
4. Lubianca Neto JF, Fuchs FD, Facco SR, et al. Is epistaxis evidence of end-organ damage in patients with hypertension? Laryngoscope. 1999;109:1111.
5. Middleton PM. Epistaxis. Emerg Med Australas. 2004;16:428.
6. Mudunuri RK, Murthy MA. The Treatment of Spontaneous Epistaxis: Conservative vs Cautery. J Clin Diagn Res. 2012;6:1523.
7. Pallin DJ, Chng YM, McKay MP, et al. Epidemiology of epistaxis in US emergency departments, 1992 to 2001. Ann Emerg Med. 2005;46:77.
8. Schaitkin B, Strauss M, Houck JR. Epistaxis: Medical versus surgical therapy: A comparison of efficacy, complications, and economic considerations. Laryngoscope. 1987;97:1392.
9. Schlosser RJ. Clinical practice. Epistaxis. N Engl J Med. 2009; 360:784.
10. Viehweg TL, Roberson JB, Hudson JW. Epistaxis: Diagnosis and treatment. J Oral Maxillofac Surg. 2006;64:511.

Phlebotomy/Venipuncture

Farrag S

OBJECTIVES

- Know the preferred venous access sites
- Understand the indications for phlebotomy
- Recognize complications of phlebotomy
- Proper equipment selection for phlebotomy
- Know to prepare the needle holder
- Describe procedural steps for fingerstick and heelstick

INTRODUCTION/BACKGROUND

- After you have performed enough **venipuncture procedures**, they tend to become quite routine
- When you are just beginning your phlebotomy training, and have never drawn blood from a live person, it can be intimidating
- It can be distilled down into a relatively straight-forward, step-by-step process.

UNIVERSAL PRECAUTIONS

- Wear gloves and a lab coat or gown when handling blood/body fluids
- Change gloves after each patient and also when contaminated
- Wash hands frequently
- Dispose of items in appropriate containers
- Place blood collection equipment away from children and psychiatric patients.

OBTAIN INFORMED CONSENT

- Introduce yourself to the patient
- Explain the procedure to the patient and gain informed consent to continue
- It is also worth explaining that the needle stick may cause some discomfort but that it will be short lived.

INDICATIONS

- Diagnostic
  - Draw blood for tests, to prepare for transfusions
  - Draw blood for blood donations
- Therapeutic
  - Routine phlebotomies for polycythemia.

CONTRAINDICATIONS TO SITES

- Extensive scars from burns and surgery
- The arm on the side of a mastectomy
- Hematoma or edema
- IV in the same extremity
  - Turn off the IV for at least 2 minutes
  - Select a vein other than the one with the IV
  - Discard the first 5 mL off the vein
  - Withdraw blood slowly
- Cannula/fistula/heparin lock.

COMPLICATIONS

- Hematoma
- Hemolysis
- Hemoconcentration
- Accidental arterial stick
- Syncope or dizziness.

BASIC EQUIPMENT

- Gloves
- An alcohol wipe
- Tourniquet
- Needle
- Needle holder
- Appropriate sample tubes
- Gauze and adhesive tape
- A sharps bin.

SITES

- Arteries pulsate, veins do not
- Most common sites
  - Median cubital and cephalic veins
- Alternate sites
  - Basilic vein or dorsal hand veins

- Last resort
  - Foot veins.

PREPARATION

- Collect equipment
- Label tubes
- Assemble needle and vacuum tube holder without piercing the tube
- Place the tube into the holder
- Position the arm for vein identification
- Select the vein.

PROCEDURE STEPS

- Place tourniquet 3–4" above site
- Palpate then clean the site
- Remove cap from needle
- Place tension on the skin 1–2" below site
- Insert the needle, bevel up, into the skin
- Push tube all the way onto the needle
- When tubes collected, release tourniquet
- Remove needle, gauze and tape patient
- If no blood was obtained
  - Change the position of the needle
    - Move it forward, backward or adjust angle
  - Loosen the tourniquet
  - Try another tube
  - Re-anchor the vein
  - Have the patient make a fist and flex
  - Prewarm the vein
  - Have the patient drink fluids if possible
- If blood stops flowing
  - The vein may have collapsed
    - Re-secure the tourniquet to increase venous filling
    - If this is not successful, remove the needle, take care of the puncture site, and redraw
  - The needle may have pulled out of the vein when switching tubes
    - Prevent this by anchoring and firmly maintaining needle position.

SPECIMEN ANALYSIS

- The proper order of draw is:
  1. Blood culture vials or bottles, sterile tubes
  2. Coagulation tube (light blue top)
  3. Serum tube (red or gold)

4. Heparin tube (green top)
5. Ethylenediaminetetraacetic acid, (EDTA) (lavender top)
6. Glycolytic inhibitor (gray top)
- After drawing the specimen, mix the tubes and get the tubes to the lab.

ALTERNATIVES TO VENIPUNCTURE

- Fingerstick
  - Middle or ring finger of nondominant hand
  - Do not use the tip or side of the finger
  - Avoid fingers that are cold, cyanotic, swollen, scarred or that have a rash
  - Discard first few drops of blood
  - Collect blood
  - Use gauze to put pressure on stick site
- Heelstick
  - Used primarily in infants
  - Prewarm the heel to increase blood flow
  - Puncture the side of the heel
  - Discard the first drop
  - Collect the blood into capillary or microcollection devices
  - Cotton or gauze over the puncture site.

SELF-ASSESSMENT QUIZ

1. Why is there a proper order for collection of multiple tubes?
   a. To make sure the most important lab is drawn first
   b. To prevent additive contamination
   c. To create one more thing you have to remember
   d. To help keep track of what lab has already been drawn
2. Which of the following is not a potential complication of venipuncture?
   a. Hematoma   b. Hemolysis
   c. Hemoconcentration   d. Accidental arterial stick
   e. None of the above   f. All of the above
3. What is the least preferred site for venipuncture?
   a. Median cubital   b. Basilic vein
   c. Dorsal hand veins   d. Foot veins
4. What is the proper order for collecting the following tubes? 1. Blood culture; 2. Glycolytic inhibitor (Gray); 3. Heparin (Green top); 4. Serum (Red top)
   a. 1 – 2 – 3 – 4   b. 1 – 3 – 2 – 4
   c. 1 – 4 – 3 – 2   d. 1 – 3 – 4 – 2
5. Which is not an indication for using phlebotomy techniques besides venipuncture?
   a. Need for a large amount of blood   b. Need for a small amount of blood
   c. Infants   d. Newborns

Answers

1. b   2. e   3. d   4. c   5. a

SUGGESTED READING

1. Baskett PJF, Dow A, Nolan J, Maull K. Practical procedures in anaesthesia and critical care. London: Mosby, 1984. p. 8-13.
2. Bhende MS. Venepuncture and peripheral venous access. In: Henreting FM, King C, (Eds) Textbook of paediatric emergency procedures. Baltimore: Williams & Wilkins, 1997. p. 803.
3. Czepizak CA, O'Callaghan JM, Venus B, Gravestein N. Vascular access. In: Kirby RR, Gravestein N, eds, Clinical anaesthesia practice. WB Saunders, Philadelphia. 1994. p. 547.
4. Datta S, Hanning CD. How to insert a peripheral venous cannula. Br J Hosp Med. 1990;43:67-9.
5. Dudley HAF, Eckersley JRT, Paterson-Brown. A guide to practical procedures in medicine and surgery. Oxford: Heinemann Medical Books. 1989. p. 48.
6. Garza D, Becan-Mcbride K. Phlebotomy handbook. Stamford, CT, USA: Appleton and Lange, 1996. p. 134.
7. Kiechle FL. So You're Going to Collect a Blood Specimen: An Introduction to Phlebotomy, 13th Edition, College of American Pathologists, Northfield, IL. 2010.
8. Lippi G, Salvagno GL, Montagnana M, Franchini M, Guidi GC. Phlebotomy issues and quality improvement in results of laboratory testing. Clin Lab. 2006;52(5-6):217-30.
9. Liu PL. Atlas of basic anaesthesia procedures. In: Barnet J, (ed). Principles and procedures in anaesthesiology, Part VI. Philadelphia: Lippincott. 1992. p. 381.
10. Roberts GH, Carson J. Venepuncture tips for radiological technologists. Radiol Technol. 1993;65:107-15.

Peripheral IV Access/Staring an IV Line

Farrag S

OBJECTIVES

- Determine concepts of fluid flow
- Understand the indications for peripheral IV access
- Be able to list the contraindications for peripheral IV access
- Equipment needed for the procedure
- Know to prepare the IV line
- Describe procedural steps for peripheral IV access
- Know steps in discontinuing a peripheral IV

INTRODUCTION/BACKGROUND

- The rate of fluid flow is proportional to radius of the cannula to the power of four, and inversely proportional to length
  - Fluids run fastest through a shorter and larger diameter tube
- Also note that the smaller the gauge of a needle, the larger its diameter
  - A 14 gauge needle has a larger diameter than a 21 gauge needle.

UNIVERSAL PRECAUTIONS

- Gloves must be worn while starting an IV
- Evaluate the need for face and eye protection as well as a gown
- IV catheters should either go into the patient or into an appropriate sharps container
- Recapping needles, putting catheters back into their sheath or dropping sharps to the floor should be strictly avoided.

OBTAIN INFORMED CONSENT

- Introduce yourself to the patient
- Explain the procedure to the patient and gain informed consent to continue
- It is also worth explaining that cannulation may cause some discomfort but that it will be short lived.

INDICATIONS

- Gain access to the peripheral circulation of a patient
  - Enables you to sample blood
  - Infuse fluids and IV medications
- For the trauma patient
  - At least two large bore (14–16G) IV catheters are usually inserted
- Critically ill patients require IV access in anticipation of future potential problems.

SITE CONTRAINDICATIONS

- Risk for fluid extravasation or low flow
  - Extremities that have massive edema, burns or injury; use other IV sites
- For the patient with abdominal trauma
  - Start the IV in an upper extremity
- For the patient with cellulitis
  - Avoid the area of infection
- Avoid an extremity with an AV fistula or on the same side of a mastectomy.

COMPLICATIONS

- The main complications of an IV catheter
  - Infection at the site
  - Development of superficial thrombophlebitis
- It is also common for the IV sites to leak interstitially.

BASIC EQUIPMENT

- Gloves and protective equipment
- Appropriate size catheter 14–25 gauge
- Non-latex tourniquet
- Alcohol swab/cleaning instrument
- Nonsterile 2 × 2 gauze
- 6 × 7 cm transparent dressing
- 3 pieces of tape approximately 10 cm long
- IV bag with prepared tubing
- Sharps container.

SITES

- Begin at a periphery of the arm
  - Veins of the forearm
  - Median cubital vein

- If a difficult stick, the veins of the dorsum of the foot or the saphenous vein of the lower leg can be used
- In circumstances in which no peripheral IV access is possible a central IV can be started.

PREPARATION

- Remove protective caps
  - From the fluid bag, and
  - The spiked end of the IV tubing
- Insert the spiked end of the IV tubing into the receptacle on the IV bag
  - While holding the IV bag inverted
- Hold the bag upright to fill the chamber
- Hang the bag from the IV pole above the patient, and open the regulating clamp.

PROCEDURE STEPS

- Don gloves and apply tourniquet
- Palpate the vein, then cleanse the site
- Prepare and inspect the catheter
- Stabilize the vein and tense the skin
- Insert the stylet through the skin
- Pull only the needle back
- Advance the catheter into the vein
- Remove the tourniquet
- Secure the catheter and attach the IV line.

USE OF ULTRASOUND TO ASSIST

- The use of a transversely oriented 7.5 MHz linear transducer is helpful to locate superficial veins
- A hand-held Doppler can be used to identify forearm veins larger than 2 mm in diameter in patients with invisible and impalpable veins, in the presence of a venous tourniquet.

REMOVAL

- Shut off the IV by closing the roller camp
- Remove the tape and transparent dressing from the tubing and catheter
- Place a nonsterile 2 × 2 gauze over the IV site and remove the catheter from the arm
- Secure the gauze in place with a piece of tape.

SELF-ASSESSMENT QUIZ

1. What is the most important factor in determining the maximum flow of the IV?
   a. Length of cannula
   b. Diameter of cannula
   c. Type of fluid
   d. All of the above

2. Which line has the highest maximum flow rate?
   a. Peripherally inserted central catheter
   b. 21 gauge peripheral IV
   c. 18 gauge peripheral IV
   d. Single lumen central catheter

3. What is not considered to be a complication of IV insertion?
   a. Infection at the site
   b. Intravenous leak
   c. Superficial thrombophlebitis
   d. Interstitial leak

4. Which site is the best initial choice for IV insertion?
   a. Veins of the forearm
   b. Dorsum of the foot
   c. Median cubital vein
   d. Saphenous vein

5. Which is not a contraindication for placement of an IV site?
   a. Burned limb
   b. Contralateral to a mastectomy
   c. Arm with cellulitis
   d. Extremity with an AV fistula

Answers

1. b   2. d   3. b   4. a   5. b

SUGGESTED READING

1. Advanced Trauma Life Support Course for Physicians. Chicago: American College of Surgeons; 1993. p. 109.

2. Baskett PJF, Dow A, Nolan J, Maull K. Practical procedures in anaesthesia and critical care. London: Mosby; 1984. p. 8-13.

3. Clutton-Brock TH. How to set up a drip and keep it going. Br J Hosp Med. 1984;32:162-7.

4. Dudley HAF, Eckersley JRT, Paterson-Brown S. A guide to practical procedures in medicine and surgery. Oxford: Heinemann Medical Books; 1989. p. 48.

5. Garza D, Becan-Mcbride K. Phlebotomy handbook. Stamford, CT, USA: Appleton and Lange; 1996. p. 134.

6. Jaques PF, Mauro MA, Keefe B. Ultrasound guidance for vascular access. J Vasc Intervent Radiol. 1992;3:427-30.

7. Statter MB. Peripheral and central venous access. Semin Paediatric Surgery. 1992;1:181-7.

8. Tager IB, Ginsberg MB, Ellis SE, et al. An epidemiological study of the risks associated with peripheral venous catheters. Am J Epidemiology. 1983;118:839-51.

9. Whiteley MS, Chang BP, Marsh H P, Williams AR, Marton HC, Horrocks M. Use of hand-held Doppler to identify 'di Y cult' forearm veins for cannulation. Ann R Coll Surg Engl. 1995;77:224-6.

Nasogastric Tube Insertion

Farrag S

OBJECTIVES

- Determine concepts of nasogastric (NG) tube use
- Understand the indications for placement of NG tube
- List the contraindications for NG tube
- List the equipment needed for the placement of NG tube
- Know how to prepare the patient for NG tube placement
- Know the procedural steps and
- Steps in discontinuing an NG tube

INTRODUCTION/BACKGROUND

- NG tubes serve both therapeutic and diagnostic purposes to gain access to GI contents
- Intended for short-term use, usually 48–72 hours
- Is a very common bedside procedure, but not without its risks.

UNIVERSAL PRECAUTIONS

- Always wear gloves
- Face and eye protection, and gown
  - Risk of vomiting.

OBTAIN INFORMED CONSENT

- Introduce yourself to the patient
- Explain the procedure to the patient and gain informed verbal consent to continue
- Explain that the patient may experience momentary discomfort such as coughing, gagging or tearing but it is essential to swallow to ease tube insertion.

INDICATIONS

- Empty the GI tract
  - Drain gastric contents
  - Obtain gastric content specimens
  - Decompression
  - Drug overdosage, presurgical, assess bleeding
  - Treat gastric immobility
  - Treat bowel obstruction
  - Prevention of vomiting and aspiration
- Initial enteral feeding or medications.

CONTRAINDICATIONS

- Severe facial trauma
- Esophageal defects
  - Strictures, varices, diverticula
- Cribiform plate disruption
  - May insert tube intracranially.

COMPLICATIONS

- Aspiration
- Tissue trauma
- Induce gagging or vomiting
  - Be prepared with suctioning.

BASIC EQUIPMENT

- NG tube
- 60 mL syringe, pH testing strip
- Water-soluble lubricant
- Xylocaine spray
- Adhesive tape and/or tube holder
- Suction device
- Stethoscope
- Cup of water/ice chips
- Emesis basin.

COMMON NASOGASTRIC TUBES

- Levin
  - Flexible soft rubber or plastic
  - Single lumen with holes distal and at the tip
  - Not used for suctioning

- Salem sump
  - Firm plastic
  - Two lumens with holes distal and at the tip
  - Second lumen serves as an air vent

PREPARATION

- Determine most patent nare
  - Through visualization or by checking airflow
- Position the patient
  - High Fowler's position (upright at 90 degrees)
  - Cover chest
- Determine NG tube length
  - Nose to earlobe, down to xiphoid process.

PROCEDURE STEPS

- Lubricate the tube, coiling the tip
- Insert tip through nare
- Advance slowly past soft palate
- Tube must turn downward into esophagus
- Swallow once tube is in esophagus
- Advance tube to mark
- Check placement—pH test or chest X-ray
- Secure the tube.

NASOGASTRIC TUBE MONITORING

- Confirm intragastric positioning
- Prevent tissue complications
- Monitor for gastric distension
- Monitor output
- Monitor vital signs.

USE OF ICE TO ASSIST IN PLACEMENT

- Partially prefreezing the tube can ease its passage
  - Prepare an ice bath
  - Curl the NG tube and place it in the bath
  - Get prepared and position the patient
  - Remove tube from bath, curl lasts 45 seconds.

REMOVAL

- Put on gloves
- Turn off the suction
- Disconnect from any devices
- Drape patient with a towel
- Remove tape
- Withdraw the tube
- Provide oral care.

SELF-ASSESSMENT QUIZ

1. A patient has an NG tube in place for 24 hours. Which finding indicates the tube is in the stomach?
   - a. Nausea
   - b. Absent bowel sounds
   - c. Tube aspirate of 7 pH
   - d. X-ray shows tip below the pylorus
2. If the NG tube is not properly suctioning, which intervention is not appropriate?
   - a. Turn the machine to high suction if low suction is sluggish
   - b. Irrigate the tube with saline
   - c. Reposition the tube if it is not draining
   - d. Monitor the client for nausea
3. What should be done immediately after inserting an NG tube?
   - a. Flush with 20 cc sterile water
   - b. Aspirate for gastric secretions
   - c. X-ray within 24 hours
   - d. Flush with 20 cc air
4. What is the difference between the Levin and the Salem sumps tubes?
   - a. Size
   - b. Length
   - c. Number of lumens
   - d. Indications for usage
5. An NG tube is being inserted and the patient begins to gag. What action is least likely to result in proper insertion?
   - a. Pulling the tube back slightly
   - b. Instructing the patient to breathe slowly
   - c. Checking the oropharynx
   - d. Continuing advancing the tube

Answers

1. d   2. a   3. b   4. c   5. d

SUGGESTED READING

1. Bourgault AM, Halm MA. Feeding tube placement in adults: Safe verification method for blindly inserted tubes. Am J Crit Care. 2009;18(1):73-6.

2. Carlson KK. Nasogastric tube insertion, care, and removal. In: ACCN procedure manual for critical care (5th ed.). St Louis, USA: Elsevier Saunders. 2005. p. 899-906.

3. Chun DH, Kim NY, Shin YS, Kim SH. A randomized, clinical trial of frozen versus standard nasogastric tube placement. World J Surg 2009;33(9):1789-92.

4. Moharari RS, Fallah AH, Khajavi MR, Khashayar P, Lakeh MM, Najafi A. The GlideScope facilitates nasogastric tube insertion: a randomized clinical trial. Anesth Analg. 2010;110(1):115-8.

5. Munden J. Eggenberger T, et al. (Eds). Nasogastric tube insertion and removal. In Handbook of primary care procedures. Philadelphia, USA: Lippincott Williams and Wilkins, 2003. p. 318-24.

6. Pillai JB, Vegas A, et al. Thoracic complications of nasogastric tube. Review of safe practice. Interact Cardio Vasc Thorac Surg 2005;4(5):429.

7. Reichman EF, Simon RR eds. Emergency Medicine Procedures. Columbus, OH: McGraw-Hill Professional; 2004.

8. Stock A, et al. Confirming nasogastric tube position in the emergency department: pH testing is reliable. Pediatric Emergency Care. 2008;24:12,805-9.

Urethral/Bladder Catheterization

Farrag S

OBJECTIVES

- Describe insertion technique of urethral catheter
- List the indications for indwelling catheter
- Describe the complications of urethral catheterization
- Know the contraindications of urethral catheterization
- Know how to perform Foley insertion and removal while maintaining sterility

INTRODUCTION/BACKGROUND

- Catheters come with and without a balloon, and different sized balloons
  - Check how much the balloon is made to hold
- Assess the need for catheterization prior to insertion
  - Use indwelling catheters as a last resort when no other methods can be employed
- Review Foley need regularly and remove the catheter as soon as possible.

UNIVERSAL PRECAUTIONS

- Wear sterile gloves during insertion
- Evaluate the need for face and eye protection as well as a gown
- Gloves are also important to decrease risk of infection in the patient.

OBTAIN INFORMED CONSENT

- Introduce yourself to the patient
- Explain the procedure to the patient and gain informed consent to continue
- Explain that urinary catheterization is uncomfortable during the procedure, but after the Foley is placed this discomfort lessens.

INTERMITTENT VERSUS INDWELLING

- If intermittent catheterization is used, perform it at regular intervals to prevent bladder overdistension
- Consider using a portable ultrasound device to assess urine volume in patients undergoing intermittent catheterization and reduce unnecessary catheter insertions.

INDICATIONS

- For indwelling catheter
  - Acute urinary retention or bladder outlet obstruction
  - Need for accurate urine output
  - Use for selected surgical procedures
  - To assist in healing of open sacral or perineal wounds
  - Prolonged immobilization
  - To improve comfort for end of life care
- For intermittent (in and out) catheter
  - Decompress bladder (obstruction or neurogenic bladder)
  - Measurement of urinary output, residual volume
  - Obtain specimen when patient cannot void
  - Remove clots from bladder with irrigation
  - In the emergency department, catheters can be used to aid in the diagnosis of hematuria
- Catheter alternatives
  - External (condom) catheters in cooperative male patients without urinary retention or bladder outlet obstruction.
  - Intermittent catheterization
    - Preferable to indwelling urethral or suprapubic catheters in patients with bladder emptying dysfunction
    - And in children with myelomeningocele and neurogenic bladder.

Contraindications

- Only one absolute contraindication:
  - *Suspected* or *confirmed* urethral injury
  - Usually associated with pelvic trauma or pelvic fractures
- Physical findings of urethral injury:
  - Blood at urethral meatus
  - Gross hematuria (found in >90% of cases)
  - Perineal hematoma
  - "High-riding" prostate gland
- Relative contraindications
  - Urethral strictures
  - Recent urethral or bladder surgery

- – Combative or uncooperative patient
- – Hypospadias is *not* a contraindication
- Inappropriate catheter use:
  - – As a substitute for proper hygiene
  - – As a means of obtaining urine for culture or other diagnostic tests when the patient can voluntarily void
  - – For prolonged postoperative duration without appropriate indications
    - ▪ Proper indications include: Repair of urethra or contiguous structures, prolonged effect of anesthesia, etc.

COMPLICATIONS

- Short-term
  - – Inability to insert, tissue trauma, paraphimosis (rare)
- Long-term
  - – Infection, stone formation, retained catheter, bladder perforation (rare).

BASIC EQUIPMENT

- Sterile gloves
- Antiseptic solution
- Sterile drapes
- Sterile lubricant
- Foley catheter
- Forceps, cotton balls
- Tubing and collection bag
- 10 cc syringe with sterile water.

SIZES

- Catheters are sized in units called French, where one French equals 1/3 of 1 mm.
- Always use the smallest gauge:
  - – Adult (16–20 French)
  - – Child (10 French)
  - – Infant (5 French feeding tube)
- Only urological patients will need a larger gauge, which will only be used on the recommendation of the urologist.

PREPARATION

- Gather the equipment
- Place patient in supine position with legs spread and feet together, consider precleaning perineum

- Open catheterization kit
  - Prepare sterile field, apply sterile gloves
  - Check balloon for patency
  - Generously coat the distal portion (2–5 cm) of the catheter with lubricant
  - Prepare cleaning swabs for one-handed access
- Apply sterile drape.

PROCEDURE STEPS

- Part one (A) Female procedure
  - Separate labia using nondominant hand. Maintain hand position until Foley inserted
  - Using dominant hand to handle forceps, cleanse periurethral mucosa with solution
    - Cleanse anterior to posterior, inner to outer, one swipe per swab, discard away from sterile field
  - Pick up catheter with gloved (and still sterile) dominant hand. Hold end of catheter loosely coiled in palm of dominant hand
  - Identify the urinary meatus and gently insert until 1 to 2 inches beyond where urine is noted
- Part one (B) Male procedure
  - Hold the penis with nondominant hand.
  - Use dominant hand and forceps to cleanse periurethral mucosa with cleansing solution
    - Cleanse anterior to posterior, inner to outer, one swipe per swab, discard away from sterile field
  - Pick up catheter with sterile dominant hand. Hold end of catheter loosely coiled in palm
  - With nondominant hand, lift the penis to perpendicular and apply light upward traction
  - Insert catheter through the meatus to the bifurcation of the Y in the catheter.
- Part two: Male and female
  - Inflate balloon, with sterile liquid
  - Gently retract catheter until inflation balloon is snug against bladder neck
  - Connect catheter to drainage system
  - Secure catheter without line tension
  - Place drainage bag below level of bladder
  - Evaluate catheter function
    - Amount, color, odor, and quality of urine.

FINISHING CONSIDERATIONS

- Failed catheterization
  - If resistance is met, do not apply force
    - Ask patient to deep breathe and try to relax
  - If questionable that tip is in the bladder do not inflate the balloon
  - If catheterization is difficult a retrograde urethrogram (RUG) may need to be performed to determine if passage is possible
- Infection prevention
  - Maintain a sterile closed system
    - Connect the urinary catheter to a sterile closed urinary drainage system
    - Ensure that the connection is patent
    - Change the bag only as needed
    - Clean the hands and wear gloves before manipulating a catheter
    - Position the drainage bag below the patient's bladder and prevent floor contact
    - Empty the bag frequently.

SPECIMEN ASPIRATION

- Obtain urine samples aseptically
  - For larger volumes, may need to clamp drainage tube prior to obtaining sample
  - Cleanse port with alcohol and aspirate sample with luer lock and syringe.

REMOVAL

- Deflate the catheter's balloon
  - Attach a luer-tipped syringe to the balloon port
  - Gently aspirate fluid
- Remove catheter gently
  - If there is resistance, ensure balloon deflated
- Monitor output after removal to ensure patient is not retaining urine
  - If the patient does not void in 4–6 hours of removing the Foley, obtain a bedside bladder scan
  - If the bladder volume is <500 mL, stimulate bladder reflex. Continue to assess the patient and repeat the bladder scan in 2 hours if the patient has not voided
  - If the bladder volume is greater than 500 mL, catheterize for residual urine volume rather than place an indwelling Foley.

SELF-ASSESSMENT QUIZ

1. How far should the catheter be inserted in a male patient?
   a. To the bifurcation of the catheter   b. Until urine flows
   c. 1 inch beyond urine flow   d. 2 inches beyond urine flow
2. Which of the following is the most common complication of urethral catheterization?
   a. Infection   b. Stone formation
   c. Decompression   d. Bladder perforation
3. Which of the following is the best size choice combination?
   a. Adult 20 French   b. Adult 16 French
   c. Child 14 French   d. Infant 10 French
4. What techniques aid in stimulating bladder reflex?
   a. Cold water to abdomen   b. Run water
   c. Flush toilet   d. All of the above
5. Which is not a sign contraindicating Foley placement?
   a. Blood at urethral meatus   b. Enlarged prostate gland
   c. Perineal hematoma   d. "High-riding" prostate gland

Answers

1. a   2. a   3. b   4. d   5. b

SUGGESTED READING

1. Ackley BJ, Ladwig GB, Swan BA, Tucker SJ. Evidence-based nursing care guidelines: Medical surgical interventions. St. Louis: Mosby Elsevier, 2008.
2. Apisarnthanarak A, et al. Effectiveness of multifaceted hospitalwide quality improvement programs featuring an intervention to remove unnecessary urinary catheters at a tertiary care center in Thialand. Infection Control and Hospital Epidemiology. 2006;28(7):791-8.
3. Crouzet J, Bertrand X, Venier AG, Badoz M, Husson C, Talon D. Control of the duration of urinary catheterization: Impact on catheter-associated urinary tract infection. J Hosp Infect. 2007;67,253-7.
4. Gray M. What nursing interventions reduce the risk of symptomatic urinary tract infection in the patient with an indwelling catheter? J Wound Ostomy Continence Nurs Soc. 2004;31(1):3-13.
5. Lee YY, Tsay WL, Lou MF, Dai YT. The effectiveness of implementing a bladder ultrasound program in non-surgical units. J Advanc Nurs. 2006;57(2):192-200.
6. Newman DK. The indwelling urinary catheter-principles for best practice. J Wound, Ostomy Continence Nurs Soc. 2007;34(6):655-61.
7. Robinson S, et al. Development of an evidence-based protocol for reduction of indwelling urinary catheter usage. MedSurg Nursing. 2007;16(3):157-61.

Lumbar Puncture

Kassar D, Piriyawat P

OBJECTIVES

- Describe the technique of lumbar puncture
- List the indications for lumbar puncture
- Describe the complications of lumbar puncture
- Know the contraindications for lumbar puncture
- Know how to perform lumbar puncture while maintaining sterile technique

INTRODUCTION/BACKGROUND

- A lumbar puncture (LP) is frequently performed in neurology, radiology, emergency rooms and on hospital wards
- The lumbar puncture can provide information that can help differentiate benign and emergent conditions.

UNIVERSAL PRECAUTIONS

- Sterile gloves must be worn
- Sterile gown is optional
- Evaluate the need for face and eye protection.

OBTAIN INFORMED CONSENT

- Introduce yourself to the patient.
- Explain the procedure to the patient and gain informed consent to continue.
- The consent discussion should include the likelihood of a post-LP headache, risk of bleeding and infection.

INDICATIONS

- Clinical suspicion of meningitis

- To rule out subarachnoid hemorrhage
  - Analyze the cerebrospinal fluid
  - Measure the CSF pressure
- Access the intrathecal space
  - To obtain CSF, inject fluid or to administer medications into the intrathecal space
- To perform myelography.

CONTRAINDICATIONS

- Signs or symptoms of raised intracranial pressure
  - Decreased level of consciousness, focal neurologic signs and papilledema
  - May lead to uncal herniation and death
- Severe bleeding diathesis or coagulation disorder or on anticoagulation therapy
- Infection at the planned puncture site.

COMPLICATIONS

- Tonsillar herniation—can manifest as a dilating pupil, change in mental state, or Cushing (HTN, bradycardia, hypopnea)
- Post-LP headache—relatively common, begins within hours to days of the LP, made worse with moving to upright
  - Blood patch may be used to seal meninges
- Infection
- Bleeding.

BASIC EQUIPMENT

- Mask, sterile gloves and gown
- Skin prep solution, sterile towels
- Small basin
- 4 × 4 gauze sponges, sponge forceps
- Local anesthetic
- 4–5 sterile test tubes with stoppers
- 25 gauge 5/8" and 22 gauge 1.5" needles
- Spinal needles, manometer, 3 way stopcock.

SITES

- Patient positioning
  - If the patient is too ill to sit upright
    - Position in a left lateral position, with legs curled up in fetal position to maximize lumbar flexion

- ▪ The back should be close to edge of the bed
- ▪ Keep shoulders, hips and back in line with each other
- Use interspaces at or below L3-L4
  - – L3-L4, L4-L5, or L5-S1 interspaces can all be used, as the spinal cord ends at L1 in adults, thus the risk of cord damage is very small
  - – The subarachnoid space at the cauda equina contains nerve roots floating free in the CSF
  - – Nerve roots are moved aside by the needle
- L4-L5 space is largest when flexed
  - – Draw line at superior border of posterior iliac crests, will intersect L4 process.

PREPARATION

- Mark landmark with needle cap, prep area with iodine, then chlorhexidine
- Place sterile drape
- Using 1% lidocaine
  - – Infiltrate skin with 25 gauge needle
  - – Interspinous tissue with 22 gauge needle.

PROCEDURE STEPS

- Insert spinal needle into the interspace in the midline and directed slightly cephalad
  - – Advance slowly until there is a decrease in resistance or a pop as the dura is penetrated
  - – Remove the stylet and wait 2 seconds to look for CSF, if none advance 1–2 mm at a time
  - – If bone is felt, partially withdraw and reposition
- Once CSF is seen use manometer to read the opening pressure in lateral decubitus.

SPECIMEN COLLECTION

- Collect 1.5–2 cc per tube and send tubes for assessment of:
  - – Cell count
  - – Culture and gram stain
  - – Glucose and protein
  - – Cell count and differential
  - – If needed for special studies like cytology, viral cultures or HSV PCR
- Serum glucose should be checked at the same time.

REMOVAL

- Replace the stylet fully into the spinal needle before withdrawing the needle

- – This will avoid aspiration of the nerve root and subarachnoid tissue on withdrawal
- Remove the needle in one motion
- Keep a gauze ready in the opposite hand to apply pressure on the puncture site for a short time
- Then place a Band Aid at the site.

SELF-ASSESSMENT QUIZ

1. What drugs are not typically injected intrathecally?
   a. Local anesthetics
   b. Antibiotics
   c. Nonsteroidal anti-inflammatories
   d. Steroids
2. At what spinal interspace should lumbar puncture not be performed?
   a. L1-L2
   b. L2-L3
   c. L3-L4
   d. L4-L5
3. What laboratory investigation is not performed on CSF?
   a. Cell count
   b. Glucose level
   c. Lipid level
   d. Protein level
4. Which of the following are components of correct positioning?
   a. Legs curled up in fetal position
   b. Back close to edge of the bed
   c. Keep shoulders, hips and back in line
   d. All of the above
5. What is not the use of lumbar puncture?
   a. Diagnostic aspiration of CSF for analysis
   b. Diagnostic collection of CSF for analysis
   c. Therapeutic reduction of CSF for increased intracranial pressure
   d. Therapeutic removal of excess CSF for normal pressure hydrocephalus

Answers

1. c   2. a   3. c   4. d   5. a

SUGGESTED READING

1. Agrawal D. Lumbar puncture. N Engl J Med. 2007;356:424.
2. Arendt KW, Segal S. Present and emerging strategies for reducing anesthesia-related maternal morbidity and mortality. Curr Opin Anaesthesiol. 2009;22:330.
3. Gorelick PB, Biller J. Lumbar puncture. Technique, indications, and complications. Postgrad Med. 1986;79:257.
4. Hebl JR. The importance and implications of aseptic techniques during regional anesthesia. Reg Anesth Pain Med. 2006;31:311.
5. Shaikh F, Brzezinski J, Alexander S, et al. Ultrasound imaging for lumbar punctures and epidural catheterisations: Systematic review and meta-analysis. BMJ. 2013;346:f1720.
6. The diagnostic spinal tap. Health and Public Policy Committee, American College of Physicians. Ann Intern Med. 1986;104:880.
7. Thomas SR, et al. Randomised controlled trial of atraumatic versus standard needles for diagnostic lumbar puncture. BMJ. 2000;321:986-90.

Digital Rectal Examination and Anoscopy

Noriega O, Kupesic Plavsic S

OBJECTIVES

- Describe digital rectal (DRE) exam and anoscopy techniques
- List the indications for DRE and anoscopy
- Describe the complications of DRE and anoscopy
- Know the contraindications for DRE and anoscopy
- Know how to perform digital rectal exam and anoscopy

INTRODUCTION/BACKGROUND

- Digital rectal exam prior to anoscopy
  - To check for pain
  - Evaluates the pelvis: Uterus and ovaries in women, prostate gland in men
  - Evaluate the cause of rectal bleeding or a change in bowel or urinary habits
  - Evaluate masses, but rectal exam alone is not used to diagnose colorectal cancer
  - Rectal exam may not find the soft internal hemorrhoids unless thrombosed (hard feel)
- Anoscopy enables direct visualization of the last 2 inches of colon
  - This 5 cm length is also called the anal canal
- An anoscope is a short, rigid, hollow tube
  - Can contain a light source as well for better visualization
- No preparation is required to empty the colon, anoscopy can be performed at any time
  - No enemas or laxatives needed.

UNIVERSAL PRECAUTIONS

- Gloves must be worn while performing both procedures.

OBTAIN INFORMED CONSENT

- Introduce yourself to the patient
- Explain the procedure to the patient, as well as the risks and benefits
- Gain informed consent to continue.

INDICATIONS

- Digital rectal examination is indicated for
  - Hemorrhoids, prostatitis, benign prostatic hyperplasia, anal condyloma, constipation, fecal incontinence, anal fissures and inflammatory bowel disease
- Anoscopy is indicated to evaluate when a digital rectal examination is not enough
  - Anal lesions, rectal bleeding, rectal pain, and banding or injection of hemorrhoids.

CONTRAINDICATIONS

- Digital rectal examination is without absolute contraindications
  - Caution in infants and toddlers, patients with neutropenia, prostatic abscesses and/or prostatitis
- Anoscopy is contraindicated in imperforate anus, massive lower GI bleeding, anal strictures, acute perirectal abscess and/or acutely thrombosed hemorrhoids
  - Caution in patients with recent anal or rectal surgery.

COMPLICATIONS

- Digital rectal examination
  - Vasovagal syncope, which is typically treated with rest and administration of fluids
  - Disseminated infection can occur with prostatic abscess or acute prostatitis
- Anoscopy is a relatively safe procedure
  - Minor irritation of the local mucosa
  - Anal or perianal fissures
  - Minor bleeding.

BASIC EQUIPMENT

- Standard lubricating jelly
- Sterile or nonsterile gloves
- Paper towels or tissue paper
- Disposable sheet

- Light source
- Anoscope.

POSITIONING

- The most common position is the lateral decubitus position with the top leg flexed at the knee and the hip
- Other positions include:
  - The knee-shoulder (lithotomy) position, legs spread and both knees flexed
  - Dorsal lithotomy position, patient on knees, with knees tucked up under body
  - On the stomach in the prone position.

PREPARATION

- Most patients do not require analgesia
- For those unable to tolerate exam due to pain, or in cases of foreign body removal
  - 2% lidocaine jelly may be inserted into the anal canal 10 minutes prior to exam
- For complicated cases, refer to a specialist for an examination under anesthesia or admission to the hospital if indicated.

PROCEDURE STEPS

- Digital rectal examination
  - Glove, spread the buttocks and inspect
    - Anus, posterior perineum, and gluteal folds
  - Lubricate the index finger and advance through the sphincter into the rectum
  - After a few seconds, the sphincter should relax more, then advance the digit farther
    - *Note* sphincter tone, pain, palpate internal structures circumferentially to evaluate for hemorrhoids, masses, note presence of stool
  - Prostate evaluation
    - Palpation: Begin at the apex and progress toward the base to determine
      - Size, consistency, nodules, fluctuance, irregularity
    - Note the seminal vesicles, proximal to the base of the prostate
      - Can be absent in some conditions
- Anoscopy
  - Generously lubricate the anoscope

- Introduce the anoscope and advance slowly while the patient bears down
  - Maintain pressure over the obturator with the thumb to keep the obturator in place
  - If contraction of the external anal sphincter is significant, constant pressure fatigues the muscles and permits insertion
  - Once the anoscope is completely inserted, remove the obturator
- Removal of anoscope
  - As the anoscope is slowly withdrawn, the anal mucosa can be visualized over the entire circumference of the canal
    - Any debris or blood can be swabbed for analysis, if desired
  - When between perianal skin and anal canal (anal verge), spasm of the external sphincter causes rapid expulsion
  - Firm counterpressure allows slow removal.

SELF-ASSESSMENT QUIZ

1. What anatomical structure can make anoscopy insertion difficult?
   a. External anal sphincter
   b. Internal anal sphincter
   c. Levator ani
   d. Coccygeus
2. Which of these statements is true?
   a. An opaque anoscope provides the clearest view of the anal mucosa
   b. Anoscopes consist of a tapered cylinder and a solid obturator that fits inside
   c. The anoscope should always be inserted without the obturator in the cylinder
   d. The patient should never be positioned in the lateral decubitus
3. Which of the following is NOT a contraindication to anoscopy?
   a. Imperforate anus
   b. Fecal incontinence
   c. Uncooperative patient
   d. Anal fissures
4. Which of the following statements is correct?
   a. Digital rectal examination should be performed after each anoscopy
   b. Digital rectal examination should be performed before all anoscopies
   c. Digital rectal examination is only performed prior to anoscopy in extenuating circumstances
   d. All are true
5. Which of the following are indications for anoscopy?
   a. Rectal bleeding
   b. Anal pain
   c. Constipation
   d. All of the above

Answers

1. a   2. b   3. b   4. b   5. d

SUGGESTED READING

1. Alonso-Coello P, Wong RF, Kuwada SK. Other strategies for evaluating rectal bleeding in younger patients. J Fam Pract. 2005;54:688.
2. Coates WC. Anorectum. In: Marx JA, Hockberger RS, Walls RM (eds). Rosen's Emergency Medicine: Concepts and Clinical Practice. 5th ed. St Louis, Mo: Mosby; 2002;Chap 91.
3. du Toit J, Hamilton W, Barraclough K. Risk in primary care of colorectal cancer from new onset rectal bleeding: 10 year prospective study. BMJ. 2006;333:69.
4. Eslick GD, Kalantar JS, Talley NJ. Rectal bleeding: epidemiology, associated risk factors, and health care seeking behaviour: A population-based study. Colorectal Dis. 2009;11:921.
5. Simmang CL, Shires GT. Diverticular disease of the colon. In: Sleisenger and Fordtran's Gastrointestinal and liver disease: Pathophysiology, diagnosis, management, 7th ed, 2002. p. 2100.
6. Strear CM, Coates WC. Anorectal Procedures. In: Roberts JR, Hedges JR (Eds). Clinical Procedures in Emergency Medicine. 4th ed. Philadelphia, Pa: WB Saunders; 2004;Chap 46.
7. Winawer S, Fletcher R, Rex D, et al. Colorectal cancer screening and surveillance: Clinical guidelines and rationale-Update based on new evidence. Gastroenterology. 2003;124:544.

18

CHAPTER

Excision of Thrombosed External Hemorrhoids

Crawford S

OBJECTIVES

- Describe excision technique for thrombosed external hemorrhoids
- List the indications for hemorrhoid removal
- Describe the complications of hemorrhoid removal
- Be able to perform the excision of thrombosed external hemorrhoids

INTRODUCTION/BACKGROUND

- Acute swelling of the venous system distal to the dentate line may allow blood to pool and clot, which can cause an acutely thrombosed external hemorrhoid
- Conservative therapy includes stool softeners, increased fiber and fluids, warm baths and topical nifedipine
- Surgical excision provides faster resolution, has low recurrence rates.

UNIVERSAL PRECAUTIONS

- Excision is a sterile procedure and sterile gloves must be worn while performing procedure
- Evaluate the need for face and eye protection as well as a gown.

OBTAIN INFORMED CONSENT

- Introduce yourself to the patient
- Explain the procedure to the patient, as well as the risks and benefits
- Gain informed consent to continue.

INDICATIONS

- Pain onset within 48–72 hours of occurrence of thrombosis

CONTRAINDICATIONS

- Possibility the lesion may not be an external hemorrhoid
- Grade IV internal hemorrhoid associated with the external hemorrhoid
- Severe coagulopathy
- Hemodynamic instability
- Relative contraindications
  - Perianal infection, anorectal fissure, portal hypertension, inflammatory bowel disease.

COMPLICATIONS

- Bleeding—control with pressure
  - If needed, use silver nitrate
- Infection—no prophylactic antibiotics
- Stricture—avoid incising anal sphincter
- Incontinence—avoid incising anal sphincter
- Pain – ensure local anesthetic used
- Perianal skin tag—common, benign complication after incision has healed.

BASIC EQUIPMENT

- Sterile gloves, sterile drape
- Antiseptic skin solution
- 1% lidocaine with epinephrine
- 5 mL syringe, 18 G and 25 G needle
- Forceps, scissors, scalpel blade
- Silver nitrate
- Sterile packing gauze
- 4 × 4 gauze, adhesive tape, and sterile dressing.

SITES/POSITIONING

- Patient should be placed in the prone position
- Use two overlapping sheets to cover the patient's buttocks, legs and back to provide for the patient's privacy.

PREPARATION

- To expose the area, tape buttocks to draw them horizontally away from the midline
- Clean area with antiseptic, starting at the hemorrhoid and working outward
- Place direct light onto the area.

- Drape the area with sterile drapes
- Anesthetize with 2 mL lidocaine into the hemorrhoid

PROCEDURE STEPS

- With scalpel remove a fusiform-shaped section through the top of the hemorrhoid
  - Excision should be oriented radially from the anal orifice
  - Remove all clots and pack loosely with gauze
- Dress the site with 4 × 4 gauze, remove tape holding buttocks open and tape gauze in place, using buttocks to assist holding gauze in place.

FOLLOW-UP

- Patients should take 3–4 sitz baths daily at home
- Can remove packing gauze in 48 hours if did not already fall off
- Acetaminophen or ibuprofen for pain control after procedure
- Continue hydration, fiber and stool softeners for 4 weeks after procedure.

SELF-ASSESSMENT QUIZ

1. Of the options available to treat hemorrhoids, which is the fastest?
   a. Stool softeners
   b. Sitz bath
   c. Surgical excision
   d. Topical nifedipine
2. Which of the following is not a contraindication to surgical excision?
   a. Pain and discomfort
   b. Possibility that the lesion may not be an external hemorrhoid
   c. Coagulopathy
   d. Hemodynamic instability
3. Which complication can be prevented by avoiding incising the anal sphincter?
   a. Bleeding
   b. Infection
   c. Pain
   d. Stricture
4. What is the correct method of taping buttocks?
   a. Tape the buttocks open after the procedure
   b. Tape the buttocks closed before the procedure
   c. Tape the buttocks closed after the procedure
   d. None of the above
5. What interventions should continue after the procedure?
   a. Hydration
   b. Fiber
   c. Stool softeners
   d. All of the above

Answers

1. c   2. a   3. d   4. c   5. d

SUGGESTED READING

1. Acheson AG, Scholefield JH. Management of haemorrhoids. BMJ. 2008; 336(7640):380-3.
2. Alonso-Coello P, Castillejo MM. Office evaluation and treatment of hemorrhoids. J Fam Pract. 2003;52(5):366-74.
3. Arthur JD. External haemorrhoidal thrombosis: Evidence for current management. Tech Coloproctol. 2013;17(1):21-5.
4. Bassford T. Treatment of common anorectal disorders. Am Fam Physician. 1992;45:1787-94.
5. Buls JG. Excision of thrombosed external hemorrhoids. Hosp Med. 1994;30:39-42.
6. Grosz CR. A surgical treatment of thrombosed external hemorrhoids. Dis Colon Rectum. 1990;33:249-50.
7. Leibach JR, Cerda JJ. Hemorrhoids: Modern treatment methods. Hosp Med. 1991;27:53-68.
8. Schussman LC, Lutz LJ. Outpatient management of hemorrhoids. Prim Care. 1986;13:527-41.
9. Zuber, T. Hemorrhoidectomy for Thrombosed External Hemorrhoids. Am Fam Physician. 2002;65(8):1629-32.
10. Zuber TJ. Office procedures. Baltimore: Lippincott Williams & Wilkins; 1999.

Endotracheal Intubation

Ainsworth C, Morang BR

OBJECTIVES

- Describe endotracheal intubation
- Be aware of the indications for intubation
- Describe the complications of endotracheal intubation
- Know the contraindications of endotracheal intubation
- Know how to perform intubation while maintaining oxygenation

INTRODUCTION/BACKGROUND

- Being able to attain an open airway is the first principle of resuscitation
- The primary purpose is to establish and maintain a safe, stable, patent airway
- Interventions begin from noninvasive methods and advance as needed to achieve a safe and stable airway:
  - Head positioning
  - Oral/nasal airway
  - Bag-valve-mask ventilation
  - Intubation.

UNIVERSAL PRECAUTIONS

- Gloves must be worn while intubating
- Evaluate the need for face and eye protection or for a gown.

OBTAIN INFORMED CONSENT

- With an emergent need for intubation, informed consent may be waived
  - Attempt to establish the patient's desired code status at the first patient encounter

- If the situation is not emergent, explain the procedure to the patient or family and gain informed consent to continue.

INDICATIONS

- Compromised airway or anticipated compromise as in sepsis
- Altered respiratory status
  - Sedation/decreased mental status
  - Inability to protect the airway
  - Absent/decreased spontaneous ventilation
  - Decreased PO_2, increased PCO_2
  - Decreased or increased respirations.

CONTRAINDICATIONS

- Tracheal fracture or disruption
- Patient's desire not to be intubated, whether through:
  - Direct patient statement
  - Code status
  - POLST form
  - Advanced directives
  - Power of attorney, or
  - Other recognized decision maker.

COMPLICATIONS

- Hypotension, raised intracranial pressure and aspiration are expected complications
- Airway damage: Lacerations or bleeding of soft tissue, tracheal or esophageal perforations and pneumothorax
- Dental damage: Remove misplaced teeth
- Esophageal intubation: Decompress the stomach.

BASIC EQUIPMENT

- Medications—including oxygen
- Endotracheal tubes—at appropriate size
- Laryngoscopes—blade and handle
- Suction—hooked up and on
- Monitoring—blood pressure, ECG, pulse oximetry, end tidal CO_2
- Assistant—to help with rapid sequence medications, cricoid pressure, etc.

PRIOR TO INTUBATION

- Head positioning
  - Extend the head and flex the neck slightly back so the patient is "sniffing"
    - Head tilt and chin lift—nontrauma patients
    - Jaw thrust—if suspected C-spine injury, previous cervical fusion or Down's syndrome
  - Changing head position may:
    - Relieve mild anatomic airway obstructions
    - Stimulate the respiratory drive
- Airway adjuncts
  - Inserted to assist in opening an airway
  - Oral airway
    - Used in unconscious or intubated patients
    - Not to be used with mandibular fractures or reactive airway disease
  - Nasal airway
    - Used in mandibular fractures, awake patients
    - Not to be used if basal skull fractures are suspected or in pregnant women
- Bag-valve-mask ventilation
  - Provides short-term oxygenation
    - When adequate ventilation is compromised and for pre-oxygenation prior to intubation
    - Contraindicated in active vomiting, known hiatal hernia, TE fistula, or facial trauma
  - Procedure
    - Open the airway and seal the mask onto the patient's face with one hand
    - Deliver high oxygen content breaths by squeezing the bag with the other hand

RAPID SEQUENCE INTUBATION WITH ADULT DOSING

- Induction: Puts patient to sleep
  - Etomidate 0.3 mg/kg (beware in seizures)
- Neuromuscular blockade: Paralysis
  - Succinylcholine 1.5–2 mg/kg (beware in renal disease)
- After intubation: Sedation
  - Midazolam 0.05–0.15 mg/kg
- Vasopressors and resuscitation medications if needed
  - Atropine, epinephrine, phenylephrine

PROCEDURE STEPS

- Select the correct tube size
  - Average size 3 for women, size 4 for men
  - Pediatric sizes by Broselow tape or (age +16)/4
- Check the endotracheal tube's cuff for leaks by inflating and deflating the balloon
- Ensure the laryngoscope light functions
- Position the head for most open airway
- Preoxygenate the patient with mask ventilations to increase their oxygen
- Open the patient's mouth with scissoring motion of fingers of right hand
- Hold the laryngoscope in the left hand
- Place the laryngoscope blade in the right side of the mouth, sweeping the tongue out of the way
- Advance the blade to the vallecula (curved blade) or epiglottis (straight blade)
- Lift the blade to expose the vocal cords
- With the endotracheal tube in the right hand, pass the tube between the vocal cords so the cuff passes the cords
- Remove the laryngoscope and stylet
- Inflate the cuff with air and hold the tube in place at the lips
- Confirm placement in trachea with end-tidal CO_2 monitor, watch for chest expansion, listen for breath sounds
- After endotracheal intubation is confirmed
  - Initiate ventilations
  - Secure the tube in place with tape
  - Obtain a chest X-ray to confirm placement
- Bite block may be placed to decrease obstruction of the tube caused by biting.

VIDEO LARYNGOSCOPY

- Is the indirect visualization of the larynx, using a fiberoptic or digital laryngoscope to visualize the cords. The image of the cords can be displayed on a monitor
- Fiberoptic intubation uses the fiberoptic scope to visualize the cords, pass into the trachea, then advance the endotracheal tube over the scope into the airway.

REMOVAL

- Decisions regarding when to extubate are based on the patient's complete clinical picture
- Extubation is performed in a step-wise fashion to ensure the patient is ready to resume spontaneous ventilation, to decrease the need for re-intubation

SELF-ASSESSMENT QUIZ

1. What verification should be performed after intubation to confirm the position (level) of the endotracheal tube?
    - a. Gastric pH monitor
    - b. Chest X-ray
    - c. End-tidal CO_2 monitor
    - d. Arterial blood gas
2. Emergency endotracheal intubation can be performed in respiratory failure and severe illness. How is it determined that a patient needs to be intubated?
    - a. Based on the complete clinical picture
    - b. By respiratory rate alone
    - c. Any hypoxia
    - d. By results on arterial blood gas (ABG)
3. Which of the following are potential complications from endotracheal intubation?
    - a. Lacerations
    - b. Tracheal perforation
    - c. Pneumothorax
    - d. All of the above
4. Which of the following is not a correct method to determine the size of the endotracheal tube for a pediatric patient?
    - a. (Age + 16) divided by 4
    - b. Based on the size of your little finger
    - c. Broselow tape
    - d. Based on patient weight
5. Complete the following sentence: The goal of endotracheal intubation is to establish and maintain _____ airway.
    - a. Safe
    - b. Stable
    - c. Patent
    - d. Safe, stable and patent

Answers

1. b   2. a   3. d   4. b   5. d

SUGGESTED READING

1. Advanced Trauma Life Support for Doctors, 7th, American College of Surgeons 2004. p. 41.
2. Hamilton RJ. Tarascon Pocket Pharmacopoeia. Sudbury: Jones and Bartlett; 2009.
3. Kleinman ME, Chameides L, Schexnayder SM, et al. Pediatric advanced life support: 2010 American Heart Association Guidelines for Cardiopulmonary Resuscitation and Emergency Cardiovascular Care. Circulation. 2010;122:S876.
4. McGill JW, Reardon RF. Tracheal intubation. In: Roberts JR, Hedges JR (Eds). Clinical Procedures in Emergency Medicine. 5th ed. Philadelphia, Pa: Saunders Elsevier, 2009.
5. Mlinek EJ Jr, Clinton JE, Plummer D, Ruiz E. Fiberoptic intubation in the emergency department. Annals of Emergency Medicine. 1990;19(4):359-62.
6. Schneider, RE, Caro, DA. Pretreatment agents. Manual of Emergency Airway Management. Lippincott Williams & Wilkins: Philadelphia; 2004. p.185.
7. Takenaka I, Aoyama K, Iwagaki T, et al. The sniffing position provides greater occipito-atlanto-axial angulation than simple head extension: A radiological study. Canadian Journal of Anesthesia. 2007;54(2);129-33.

Thoracentesis

Crawford S

OBJECTIVES

- Describe the thoracentesis technique
- List the indications for thoracentesis
- Describe the complications of thoracentesis
- Know the contraindications for thoracentesis

INTRODUCTION/BACKGROUND

- Thoracentesis is performed to remove fluid from the pleural space between the lungs and chest wall
- There is usually only a small amount of fluid in the space. Excess fluid can be caused by many conditions such as infection, inflammation, heart failure and cancer
- Confirm presence of a pleural effusion with a chest X-ray.

UNIVERSAL PRECAUTIONS

- Sterile gloves must be worn
- Evaluate the need for face and eye protection as well as a gown.

OBTAIN INFORMED CONSENT

- Introduce yourself to the patient
- Explain the procedure to the patient, as well as the risks and benefits
- Gain informed consent to continue.

INDICATIONS

- Remove excess pleural fluid
  - Therapeutic: Relieve shortness of breath and pain
  - Diagnostic: Determine the cause of the effusion

CONTRAINDICATIONS

- Uncooperative patient
- Coagulopathy
- Portal hypertension
  - May have pleural varices and increased risk during thoracentesis.

COMPLICATIONS

- A partial collapse of the lung also known as pneumothorax
  - Occurs if the needle used to remove the pleural fluid punctures the lung, allowing air to flow into the pleural space
- Pulmonary edema
  - Occurs if a large amount of fluid is removed
- Infection and bleeding
- Damage to the liver or spleen.

BASIC EQUIPMENT

- Skin prep solution
- Sterile gloves and towels
- 18, 22 and 25 gauge needles
- 16 gauge central line, dilator and J wire
- 3-way stopcock, IV tubing with extension
- Scissors, syringe
- Vacuum bottles.

PREPARATION

- Have patient sit up straight on the edge of the bed
- Place bedside table in front of patient
  - Pillow on table, head and arms on pillow
- Percuss the back to find the fluid level
  - Locate the interspace two spaces below, but not below the 8th intercostal space
  - Mark the spot, prep and drape the area
  - Insert the needle at hemithorax midline.

PROCEDURE STEPS

- Anesthetize the skin, making a wheal
- Insert central line needle over the superior edge of the rib
  - Once over the top of the rib, advance into the chest while aspirating until pleural fluid returns
  - Draw off samples into syringe
  - Remove needle, leaving catheter in place

- Attach IV tubing to catheter and drain fluid
- Take <1 L to minimize edema.

ASPIRATE ANALYSIS

- Common tests performed on pleural fluid
    - Cell count, pH, protein, lactate dehydrogenase, glucose, amylase, gram stain, culture, and cytology

USE OF ULTRASOUND TO ASSIST

- With ultrasound guidance, probe marker should point to the head
- Locate the largest pocket of fluid and mark the location
    - Rotate the transducer to 180 to visualize the field between the ribs
- Then proceed as normal with tap.

REMOVAL

- If the fluid stops flowing, the cannula position can be adjusted slightly to attempt to get more fluid out
- Withdraw the catheter once fluid stops draining.

SELF-ASSESSMENT QUIZ

1. Which of the following is *not* a contraindication to performing thoracentesis?
    a. Herpes zoster over the proposed injection site
    b. Dyspnea
    c. Severe hemodynamic compromise
    d. Uncontrolled bleeding
2. Which of the following statements is false?
    a. The patient should be positioned at the edge of the bed, leaning forward
    b. The site of needle entry should be 1–2 spaces below the level of effusion
    c. The needle should be inserted along the superior edge of the rib
    d. The needle may be inserted at any level along the hemithorax midline
3. Which of the following is a potential complication of thoracentesis?
    a. Localized infection at the injection site
    b. Post-expansion pulmonary edema
    c. Pneumothorax
    d. All of the above
4. What are potential causes of pleural effusions?
    a. Cancer   b. Infection
    c. Bleeding   d. All of the above
5. What tests are *not* commonly checked on the fluid from a thoracentesis?
    a. Cell count   b. Protein
    c. TB   d. Lactate dehydrogenase

Answers

1. b   2. d   3. d   4. d   5. c

SUGGESTED READING

1. Blok B, Ilbrado A: Respiratory Procedures. In Roberts JR, Hedges JR, et al. (Eds). Clinical Procedures in Emergency Medicine, 4th ed. Pennsylvania, Elsevier. 2004. p. 171-186.
2. Daniels CE, Ryu JH. Improving the safety of thoracentesis. Curr Opin Pulm Med. 2011;17:232.
3. Diacon AH, Brutsche MH, Solèr M. Accuracy of pleural puncture sites: A prospective comparison of clinical examination with ultrasound. Chest. 2003;123:436.
4. Duncan DR, Morgenthaler TI, Ryu JH, Daniels CE. Reducing iatrogenic risk in thoracentesis: Establishing best practice via experiential training in a zero-risk environment. Chest. 2009;135:1315.
5. Josephson T, Nordenskjold CA, Larsson J, et al. Amount drained at ultrasound-guided thoracentesis and risk of pneumothorax. Acta Radiol. 2009;50:42.
6. Pagana KD, Pagana TJ. Mosby's Manual of Diagnostic and Laboratory Tests, 4th ed. St. Louis: Mosby; 2010.
7. Temes RT. Thoracentesis. N Engl J Med. 2007;356:641.
8. Thomsen TW, DeLaPena J, Setnik GS. Videos In Clinical Medicine: Thoracentesis. N Engl J Med. 2006;355:e16.

21

Chest Tube Placement

Olivas VJ

OBJECTIVES

- List the indications for chest tube placement
- Be able to describe chest tube placement
- Describe the complications of chest tube placement
- Know the contraindications for chest tube placement
- Know how to perform chest tube placement

INTRODUCTION/BACKGROUND

- Chest tubes (also known as thoracotomy) are used for many conditions that can compromise respiratory function
- The pleural membranes envelop the lungs and line the thoracic cavity
  - If excess air of fluid collects in the pleural space the negative pressure is affected
  - Tube thoracostomy with suction can restore negative pressure to re-expand the lung.

UNIVERSAL PRECAUTIONS

- Sterile gown and gloves to be used during insertion
- Evaluate the need for face and eye protection.

OBTAIN INFORMED CONSENT

- Introduce yourself to the patient
- Explain the procedure to the patient and gain informed consent to continue.

INDICATIONS

- Pneumothorax (not under 400 mL)
  - Ventilated patient or secondary pneumothorax
  - Any tension pneumothorax (after needle relief)
  - If recurrent or persistent pneumothorax (after aspiration)
- Malignant pleural effusion
- Empyema or parapneumonic effusion
- Traumatic hemopneumothorax
- Esophageal rupture.

CONTRAINDICATIONS

- Multiple adhesions
- Pulmonary blebs
- Immediate need for open thoracotomy
- Bleeding disorder
- Overlying skin infection.

COMPLICATIONS

- Lung laceration
- Intercostal vessels and nerve laceration
- Long thoracic nerve laceration
- Solid organ puncture
- Re-expansion pulmonary edema
- Infection: Watch drainage at dressing site
- Bleeding: Think of this if drainage exceeds 100 mL/hr or if drainage is bright red
- Mechanical problem: Kinking and clog.

UNIVERSAL PRECAUTIONS

- Sterile gown and gloves to be used during insertion
- Evaluate the need for face and eye protection

OBTAIN INFORMED CONSENT

- Introduce yourself to the patient
- Explain the procedure to the patient and gain informed consent to continue.

BASIC EQUIPMENT

- Sterile gown, gloves and drapes
- Scalpel and blade, suture set with suture

- Sterile gauze swabs, syringes and needles
- Skin antiseptic, local anesthetic
- Curved clamp for blunt dissection
- Chest drain, drainage system, suction unit and tubing
- Dressing with adhesive border.

SITES

- Stay in the safe triangle
  - Anterior border of latissimus dorsi
  - Lateral border of pectoralis major
  - Horizontal line at nipple level
- Over the rib below the fourth to fifth intercostal space at the midaxillary line
  - Pneumothorax: Aim towards apex
  - Pleural effusion: Aim towards base.

PREPARATION

- Position with affected side up
- Clean skin with antiseptic
- Drape site with sterile drapes
- Anesthetize skin, subcutaneous tissue, periosteum of rib, chest-wall muscles and pleura with 1% lidocaine
- Note: When placing sutures, make sure to place untied horizontal mattress sutures as well as the securing sutures.

PROCEDURE STEPS

- Make incision and bluntly dissect subcutaneous tissues with hemostat
- Push hemostat over top of rib into pleura
- Grasp chest tube with hemostat and advance until all holes are inside
- Suture to skin, tie, then wrap suture around tube once and tie to the tube
- Apply occlusive dressing and attach to drainage system.

REMOVAL

- Criteria
  - Drainage <10 mL/hr for 6hr preremoval
  - No air leak present
  - Stable respiratory status
  - Respiratory rate <24/min
  - No acute respiratory distress
  - Coagulation parameters within normal limits

- Supplies
  - Dressing tray with occlusive dressing
  - Chlorhexidine antiseptic solution
  - Suture cutter/scissors
  - 4 × 4 gauze
  - Nonsterile gloves
  - Tape
  - Blue pad, clamps
  - Mask and face shield
- Procedure
  - Premedicate with analgesic, discontinue suction and clamp chest tube
  - Remove dressing and sutures, clean site
  - Apply occlusive dressing and create a seal
  - Instruct patient to exhale
  - In a smooth and rapid motion, remove tube, applying occlusive dressing and pull uncut mattress suture tight
  - Obtain chest X-ray within 4 hours of removal.

SELF-ASSESSMENT QUIZ

1. Which of the following signs indicates a chest tube may be removed?
   a. Drainage is 100 mL/hr
   b. Respiratory rate is 32
   c. No acute respiratory distress
   d. Presence of an air leak
2. Chest tubes may be used for drainage in what types of situations?
   a. Pleural effusion—drains fluids
   b. Hemothorax - drains blood
   c. Pneumothorax—drains air
   d. All of the above
3. If respiratory distress occurs after the procedure and lung sounds are absent what is occurring?
   a. The tube is not working
   b. The lung is not reinflated
   c. The suction is not working
   d. The tube is in the wrong place
4. What is a contraindication to chest tube insertion?
   a. Normal platelet level
   b. INR of 3
   c. Cellulitis of contralateral chest wall
   d. Pneumothorax
5. What is an indication of fresh bleeding?
   a. Drainage of <10 mL/hr
   b. Drainage of <50 mL/hr
   c. Drainage of <100 mL/hr
   d. Drainage of >100 mL/hr

Answers

1. c   2. d   3. b   4. b   5. d

SUGGESTED READING

1. Ball CG, Lord J, Laupland KB, et al. Chest tube complications: how well are we training our residents? Can J Surg. 2007;50:450.

2. Baumann MH, Strange C, Heffner JE, et al. Management of spontaneous pneumothorax: an American College of Chest Physicians Delphi consensus statement. Chest. 2001;119:590.

3. Becker DE. Arterial catheter insertion (Perform). AACN Procedure Manual for Critical Care, 4th Ed., WB Saunders, Philadelphia, PA; 2001. p. 361-5.

4. Dalbec DL, Krome RL. Thoracostomy. Emerg Med Clin North Am. 1986;4:441.

5. Menger R, Telford G, Kim P, et al. Complications following thoracic trauma managed with tube thoracostomy. Injury. 2012;43:46.

6. Tomlinson MA, Treasure T. Insertion of a chest drain: how to do it. British Journal of Hospital Medicine 2003;58:6;248-52.

7. Vasseur BG. A simplified technique for closing thoracostomy incisions. Ann Thorac Surg. 2004;77:1467.

Paracentesis

Crawford S

OBJECTIVES

- List the indications for paracentesis
- Be able to describe the course of paracentesis
- Describe the complications of paracentesis
- Know the contraindications for paracentesis
- Know how to perform paracentesis

INTRODUCTION/BACKGROUND

- Ascites is as an abnormal collection of fluid with the peritoneal cavity.
  - Small amounts of fluid may by asymptomatic
  - Larger amounts may cause abdominal pain, nausea, anorexia and infection
- The process of aspirating fluid from the abdomen is called paracentesis
  - Done to relieve symptoms and/or to retrieve fluid samples for diagnostic testing.

UNIVERSAL PRECAUTIONS

- Sterile gloves must be worn while performing procedure
- Evaluate the need for face and eye protection as well as a gown.

OBTAIN INFORMED CONSENT

- Introduce yourself to the patient
- Explain the procedure to the patient, as well as the risks and benefits
- Gain informed consent to continue.

INDICATIONS

- Diagnostic tap is used for
    - New-onset ascites: Paracentesis obtains fluid for analysis to determine etiology, transudative vs exudative, cell cytology
    - To evaluate for suspected spontaneous or secondary bacterial peritonitis
- Therapeutic tap is used for:
    - Respiratory compromise secondary to ascites
    - To relieve abdominal pain or pressure.

CONTRAINDICATIONS

- Any acute abdomen (needs surgery)
- Severe thrombocytopenia (platelet count <20,000) may need a platelet infusion
- Coagulopathy (INR >2) may need fresh frozen plasma before the procedure
- Infections like abdominal wall cellulitis
- Caution in pregnancy, distended bowel, distended urinary bladder.

COMPLICATIONS

- Bowel or bladder perforation
- Infection—avoid with sterile procedure
- Hemodynamic compromise—from large volume fluid removal (limit to 4–5 L to prevent hypotension)
- Fluid leak—use Z tract to prevent leakage
- Sepsis.

BASIC EQUIPMENT

- Antiseptic swab sticks, fenestrated drape
- Lidocaine, 10 and 60 mL syringe
- Needles: 20, 22 and 25 gauge
- Scalpel blade, 4 × 4 gauze, tape
- Catheter, 8F, over 18 Ga × 7 1/2" needle with 3-way stopcock, self-sealing valve, and a 5 mL Luer-lock syringe
- Tubing set with clamps, drainage system, specimen vials.

SITES

- Position patients in the lateral decubitus position, as the bowel can float upward and out of the path of the needle

- Midline: 2 cm below the umbilicus in the midline, through the linea alba
- Lateral if there is midline scarring
  - 5 cm superior and medial to the anterior superior iliac spines on either side.

USE OF ULTRASOUND TO ASSIST

- A low frequency transducer in a sterile sheath is positioned sagittally
  - Infraumbilical or lateral on a supine patient
- The deepest pocket of fluid is identified
  - Needle is inserted through the abdomen
  - The tip of the needle is visualized as a hyperechoic structure
  - US guidance to avoid puncture of the moving bowel and the bladder.

PREPARATION

- Empty the patient's bladder, either voluntarily or with a Foley catheter
- Position the patient and prepare the skin around the entry site with an antiseptic solution
- Apply a sterile fenestrated drape to create a sterile field
- Use the 5 mL syringe and the 25-gauge needle to administer local lidocaine.

PROCEDURE STEPS

- Keeping an eye on the planned tract
  - Pull the skin 2 cm caudally (Z-tract)
  - Insert the needle perpendicular with slow advancement while aspirating
  - With entry to the peritoneum, ascitic fluid can be seen, then advance 5 mm further
- Advance catheter over needle
  - May use scalpel to nick skin for passage
  - Remove needle and attach 60 mL syringe to stopcock and catheter
- With syringe, aspirate to obtain ascitic fluid for analysis in a diagnostic tap
- Attach to a vacuum bottle or a drainage bag to remove large volumes for a therapeutic tap
- The catheter can become occluded so if the flow stops manipulate the catheter so flow resumes.

ASPIRATE ANALYSIS

- May include
  - Gram stain, cell count, total protein level
  - Bacterial culture

- Cytology
- Triglyceride levels
- Bilirubin level, glucose level
- Albumin level with same day serum albumin
- Amylase level
- Lactate dehydrogenase (LDH) level.

REMOVAL

- Remove the catheter after the desired amount of ascitic fluid has been drained
- Apply firm pressure to stop bleeding or leakage, if present
- Place a bandage over the puncture site.

SELF-ASSESSMENT QUIZ

1. What is an absolute contraindication for paracentesis?
   - a. Acute abdomen
   - b. Increased INR
   - c. Abdominal wall cellulitis
   - d. Pregnancy
2. Ascitic fluid laboratory analysis commonly includes which of the following?
   - a. Ascites albumin
   - b. Differential cell count
   - c. Cultures
   - d. All of the above
3. Which method is a way to decrease the likelihood of bowel perforation?
   - a. Placing the patient in Trendelenburg
   - b. Placing the patient in lateral decubitus
   - c. Ensuring the coagulation status is normal
   - d. Use "Z-tract" method with needle insertion
4. Which of the following is the best site of entry for paracentesis?
   - a. 2 cm infraumbilical, through a skin infection
   - b. 2 cm infraumbilical, through a surgical scar
   - c. Left lower quadrant, cephalad and medial to the ASIS through intact skin
   - d. Right lower quadrant, cephalad and medial to ASIS through a superficial vein
5. Which of the following is an indication for paracentesis?
   - a. Relief of symptoms of ascites
   - b. Diagnosis of peritoneal infections
   - c. Evaluation of type of ascites
   - d. All are indications for paracentesis

Answers

1. a   2. d   3. b   4. c   5. d

SUGGESTED READING

1. Duggal P, Farah KF, Anghel G, Marcus RJ, Lupetin AR, Babich MM, et al. Safety of paracentesis in inpatients. Clin Nephrol. 2006;66(3):171-6.
2. Glickman RM, Isselbacher KJ. Abdominal swelling and ascites. Harrison's Principles of Internal Medicine, 13th ed. New York, McGraw-Hill; 1994, p. 234.
3. Kuiper JJ, van Buuren HR, de Man RA. Ascites in cirrhosis: a review of management and complications. Neth J Med. 2007;65(8):283-8.
4. McGibbon A, Chen GI, Peltekian KM, van Zanten SV. An evidence-based manual for abdominal paracentesis. Dig Dis Sci. 2007;52(12):3307-15.
5. Reichman E, Simon RR. Emergency Medicine Procedures. 1st. New York, NY: McGraw-Hill Professional; 2003.
6. Roberts JR, Hedges JR. Clinical Procedures in Emergency Medicine, 4th ed. Pennsylvania: Elsevier; 2004, p. 851-6.
7. Wong CL, Holroyd-Leduc J, Thorpe KE, Straus SE. The rational clinical examination: Does this patient have bacterial peritonitis or portal hypertension? How do I perform a paracentesis and analyze the results? JAMA. 2008;299(10):1166-78.

Arterial Lines

Ainsworth C, Morang BR

OBJECTIVES

- List the indications for arterial lines placement
- Describe insertion technique
- Describe the complications of arterial lines
- Know the contraindications for arterial lines placement
- Know how to perform arterial cannulation

INTRODUCTION/BACKGROUND

- Arterial lines are used
  - For collection of blood and for invasive arterial blood pressure measurement
  - In intensive care units and intraoperatively
  - Are the gold standard for accurate blood pressure measurements
- The radial artery is the preferred site for insertion.

UNIVERSAL PRECAUTIONS

- Sterile gloves must be worn while inserting arterial line
- Evaluate the need for face and eye protection as well as a gown.

OBTAIN INFORMED CONSENT

- Introduce yourself to the patient
- Explain the procedure to the patient, as well as the risks and benefits
- Gain informed consent to continue.

INDICATIONS

- Need for continuous blood pressure measurements
  - Hemodynamically unstable patients receiving ionotropic agents
  - Patients with severe cardiovascular disease undergoing surgery

- Frequent arterial blood gas analysis
  - In patients with respiratory failure
  - In patients with severe acid/base imbalances.

CONTRAINDICATIONS

- Failed Allen's test—determines extent of collateral perfusion in the hand
  - Compress both the radial and ulnar arteries at the same time
  - Release the ulnar artery while keeping the radial compressed
  - If hand color does not return in less than 5 seconds, this test is failed.

COMPLICATIONS

- Arterial thrombosis
  - Risk increases with decreasing wrist circumference
  - Risk increases rapidly in first 24 hours, then slowly decreases
- Occult bleeding or hematoma
- Ischemic digits
  - Remove catheter and monitor the digit.

BASIC EQUIPMENT

- Chloraprep, betadine or alcohol prep
- Tape, arm board, sterile gloves and towels
- Lidocaine, syringe and 25 gauge needle
- 20 gauge angiocatheter
- 2-0 silk sutures and needle driver
- Pressure bag, IV tubing, 500 mL saline
- Monitoring wires, stopcock.

SITES

- In order of most preferred to least preferred
  - Radial: Low complication rates, superficial artery that can be easily compressed
  - Femoral
  - Dorsalis pedis
  - Axillary
    - Can also use ulnar, brachial, posterior tibial arteries.

PREPARATION

- Perform Allen's test prior to beginning
- Position patient's wrist and hand
  - Expose the ventral surface of the arm
  - Dorsiflex wrist over a rolled towel
  - Secure the palm and upper forearm to arm board with tape

- Palpate radial pulse and mark location
- Sterile prep wrist with chloraprep, betadine or alcohol
- Apply lidocaine 2 mL under skin of area
- Draw up 5 mL of saline
  - Flush IV catheter with saline.

PROCEDURE STEPS

- With the angiocatheter needle angled 45 degrees toward arm
  - Enter skin just distal to palpated artery site
  - Slowly advance needle until blood returns
- Slowly advance the guide wire into artery
  - Do not force the wire, be smooth and gentle
- Compress artery and remove needle
- Advance cannula over top of guidewire
- Remove guidewire
- Attach flush syringe with stopcock
  - Reflush cannula with 2 cc saline
  - Turn stopcock to seal artery
  - Remove syringe
- Connect transducer and high-pressure infusion set to stopcock
- Consider removing arm board or towel
- Secure the catheter to the skin with sutures and cover with a sterile dressing

MONITORING ARTERIAL LINE

- Set up invasive blood pressure monitoring
  - Waveforms show peak systolic pressure, pulse pressure, mean arterial pressure
  - Place transducer at level of right atrium
- In case of poor arterial waveform
  - Check line connections and stopcock
  - Check that wrist is dorsiflexed
  - Ensure arm is not elevated
  - Ensure good blood return.

REMOVAL

- Disconnect the line from the monitor
- Clamp the T-piece
- Take out the sutures, pull the catheter and compress the site with a sterile 4 × 4 for 3–5 minutes
- Place a compression dressing, then ensure the hand is still perfused
- Recheck the site hourly for a few hours.

SELF-ASSESSMENT QUIZ

1. What arteries can be used for the placement of an arterial line besides the radial artery?
   a. Ulnar
   b. Axillary
   c. Dorsalis pedis
   d. All of the above

2. How do you know that the patient's hand will not be at risk following a radial artery line placement?
   a. The hand does not turn pale during Allen's test
   b. The hand pinks up when radial artery released
   c. The hand pinks up with release of the ulnar artery
   d. The hand stays pale after Allen's test

3. Which of the following are complications of arterial line insertion?
   a. Thrombosis
   b. Hematoma
   c. Infection
   d. All of the above

4. What is the correct level for the transducer?
   a. At the wrist
   b. At the waist
   c. At the shoulder
   d. At the right atrium

5. What are arterial lines used for?
   a. Blood pressure monitoring
   b. Blood draws
   c. Arterial blood gas monitoring
   d. All of the above

Answers

1. d   2. c   3. d   4. d   5. d

SUGGESTED READING

1. Cousins T, O'Donnel J. Arterial Cannulation: A Critical Review. AANA Journal. 2004;72:4:267-71.
2. Durbin CG Jr. Radial arterial lines and sticks: what are the risks? Respir Care. 2001;46:229-30.
3. Frezza EE, Mezghebe H. Arterial catheter use in surgical or medical intensive care units: An analysis of 4932 patients. Am Surg. 1998;64:127-31.
4. Gardner RM. Direct blood pressure measurement – dynamic response requirements. Anesthesiology. 1981;54(3):227-36.
5. McGregor AD. The Allen test: An investigation of its accuracy by fluorescein angiography. J Hand Surg [Br]. 1987;12:82-5.
6. Pauca AL, Wallenhaupt SL, Kon ND, Tucker WY. Does radial artery pressure accurately reflect aortic pressure? Chest. 1992;102:1193-8.
7. Scheer B, Perel A, Pfeiffer UJ. Clinical review: Complications and risk factors of peripheral arterial catheters used for haemodynamic monitoring in anaesthesia and intensive care medicine. Crit Care. 2002;6(3):199-204.
8. Ward M, Langton JA. Blood pressure management. Contin Educ Anaesth Crit Care Pain. 2007;7(4):122-6.

Central Venous Catheterization

Ainsworth C

OBJECTIVES

- List the indications for placement of central venous lines
- Describe procedural steps for central venous lines placement
- Describe the complications of central venous lines
- Know the contraindications for central venous lines
- Know how to perform central vein cannulation while maintaining sterility

INTRODUCTION/BACKGROUND

- Always attempt to place peripheral IV prior to central line placement
  - Attempt to place least invasive lines first
- The decision to place the central venous catheter has several points to consider
  - Site choice: Jugular, subclavian or femoral
  - Catheter choice: By lumen number or type
- Purpose of catheter has a large effect on catheter type and site choice.

UNIVERSAL PRECAUTIONS

- This is a sterile procedure
- Gloves, gown, mask must be worn during insertion
- Evaluate the need for eye protection.

OBTAIN INFORMED CONSENT

- Introduce yourself to the patient
- Explain the procedure to the patient, as well as the risks and benefits
- Gain informed consent to continue.

INDICATIONS

- Need for central venous pressure monitoring
- Need for reliable venous access
- Poor peripheral access
- Need for large volume resuscitation
- Administration of inotropic medication or TPN

CONTRAINDICATIONS

- Coagulopathy
  - INR >1.5
  - Platelets <50
- Venous thrombosis
- Untreated sepsis.

COMPLICATIONS

- Internal jugular
  - Carotid cannulation, infection, pneumothorax air embolus, malposition, dysrhythmia
- Subclavian
  - Artery cannulation, pneumothorax, infection, air embolus, malposition
- Femoral
  - Artery cannulation, infection, patient must stay flat while line is in.

BASIC EQUIPMENT

- Sterile gown/gloves/mask/hat and drape
- Chloraprep
- Ultrasound with sterile probe cover
- Appropriate line kit
- Lidocaine, flush, dressing (usually in kit)
- Nurse for assistance
- Monitors (ECG and pulse ox)
- End pieces for catheter.

LINE TYPES

- Triple lumen catheter: 6 g and 2 × 18 g
- Double Lumen Catheter: 14 g and 16 g
- Cordis: 7.5F, rapid volume, Swan-Ganz
- Groshong: Plasmapheresis or dialysis

- Mehurkur: Dialysis
- Hohn catheter: Tunneled line
- Hickman: Tunneled line, 1-2 lumen
- Port-A-Cath: Tunneled, subcutaneous port.

SITES

- Subclavian vein—highest risk of line malposition
- Internal jugular vein—contraindicated in patients with increased intracranial pressure
- Femoral vein—contraindicated in patients with severe abdominal trauma, highest risk of venous thrombosis, last choice unless there is ongoing CPR.

PREPARATION

- Gather equipment and place flush in tray
- Position patient and prep skin
  - Positioning for subclavian
    - Place patient supine in Trendelenburg position
    - Hyperextend back with towel roll under thoracic spine
    - Turn patient head away
    - Place traction on ipsilateral arm
    - Aim needle from distal third of clavicle toward sternal notch
  - Positioning for internal jugular
    - Supine in 15 degrees Trendelenburg
    - Hyperextend the neck and turn head away
    - Palpate sternal and clavicular muscle heads of the sternocleido-mastoid
      - Needle should enter between the muscle heads, lateral to the carotid artery
      - Insert needle at 30 degree angle to skin and aim toward ipsilateral nipple
      - Best practice: Use ultrasound
  - Positioning for femoral
    - Position the patient supine, flat
    - Flex and abduct hip
    - Locate femoral pulse just distal to inguinal crease by placing finger on femoral artery
    - Insert needle at 30 degree angle to skin medial to pulse, aiming at the umbilicus (location should be 2–3 cm distal from inguinal ligament)
- Put on sterile gear, place full body drape
- Anesthetize area with lidocaine

- Prepare line by flushing all ports
- Place equipment on field in easy reach
- Loosely attach insertion needle to 5 cc syringe.

PROCEDURE STEPS

- Puncture skin and advance catheter while aspirating. When blood return occurs, remove syringe and insert guidewire through needle 1/2 to 3/4 the length of the wire. Do not force the wire
- Remove needle-holding guidewire firmly
  - Never let go of the wire
- Enlarge the entry site with a small dilator
  - May need to make a skin nick with blade
- Slide catheter over the wire into vein with a twisting motion until hub is at the skin
- Remove the guidewire
- Secure catheter with sutures
- Attach IV tubing
- Apply sterile dressing
- For IJ or subclavian line, obtain CXR to rule out a pneumothorax. Femoral vein on the left, obtain abdominal XR to confirm that the line is in the vena cava.

PROCEDURAL TIPS

- If arterial (pressure >30): withdraw needle and hold extended pressure
- If no venous blood is obtained withdraw needle, re-aim and try again
- Three attempts are maximum by one provider
- A CXR must be obtained after IJ or SVC line placement or even line attempt
- Conversion of cordis to triple lumen catheter (TLC) or removal before the patient leaves to the ICU.

REMOVAL

- Use sterile scissors or suture removal kit
- Remove catheter dressing and sutures
- For IJ or subclavian catheter, have the patient take a deep breath in and hold it in
- Withdraw the catheter fairly quickly then apply pressure with a sterile antibiotic ointment gauze pad until bleeding stops
- Ensure the entire catheter was removed
- Apply a sterile, air-occlusive dressing.

SELF-ASSESSMENT QUIZ

1. What is the least preferred site in patients with elevated intracranial pressure?
   a. Internal jugular   b. External jugular
   c. Subclavian   d. Femoral

2. What is the sign that an artery has been accessed instead of a vein?
   a. Dark blood   b. Pressure >30
   c. Pressure <30   d. Absence of blood

3. What is the chest X-ray following central line placement looking for?
   a. Pneumothorax   b. Position of tip of catheter
   c. Confirmation vein was cannulized   d. A and B
   e. All of the above

4. What central line catheter is the best choice for a patient in need of large volume fluid resuscitation?
   a. Triple lumen catheter   b. Double lumen catheter
   c. Cordis   d. Hickman catheter

5. Which of the following is an indication for a central venous catheter?
   a. Septic shock patient   b. Planned coronary angiogram
   c. Administration of vasopressors   d. Initiation of IV antibiotics

Answers

1. c   2. b   3. d   4. c   5. a

SUGGESTED READING

1. Boyd R, Saxe A, Phillips E. Effect of patient position upon success in placing central venous catheters. Am J Surg. 1996;172:380.

2. Higgs ZC, Macafee DA, Braithwaite BD, Maxwell-Armstrong CA. The Seldinger technique: 50 years on. Lancet. 2005;366:1407.

3. Kost, SI. Ultrasound-assisted venous access. In: Textbook of Pediatric Emergency Procedures, 2nd edition, King, C, Henretig, FM (Eds), Lippincott Williams and Wilkins: Philadelphia; 2008. p.1255.

4. McGee et al. Articles: Preventing Complications of Central Venous Catheters. NEJM. 2003;348;121123-33

5. Polderman KH, Girbes AJ. Central venous catheter use. Part 1: Mechanical complications. Intensive Care Med. 2002;28:1.

6. Timsit JF. Central venous access in intensive care unit patients: is the subclavian vein the royal route? Intensive Care Med. 2002;28:1006.

Peripherally Inserted Central Catheter

Hardin NB

- List the indications for peripherally inserted central catheter (PICC)
- Describe insertion technique of PICC
- Describe the complications of PICC
- Know the contraindications and considerations for PICC
- Be able to perform procedure while maintaining sterile technique

INTRODUCTION/BACKGROUND

- The peripherally inserted central catheter is a long, thin line that can stay in place up to 12 months for blood sampling, medication administration and total parenteral nutrition (TPN)
- It allows central venous access through a peripheral vein and is less invasive than a central catheter
- Is inserted through the basilic or cephalic veins and advanced to the subclavian.

UNIVERSAL PRECAUTIONS

- Mask
- Sterile gown
- Sterile gloves
- Hair cover/cap
- Sterile drapes
- This is a sterile procedure to reduce the risk of contamination and decrease the likelihood of future catheter-related infections.

OBTAIN INFORMED CONSENT

- Introduce yourself to the patient
- Explain the procedure to the patient, as well as the risks and benefits
- Gain informed consent to continue
- Write an informed consent note in the chart.

INDICATIONS

- Long-term intravenous access needed for medication administration
- Total parenteral nutrition administration
- Administration of solutions that may be irritating to peripheral veins.

CONTRAINDICATIONS

- With tourniquet in place, no visible or palpable upper extremity veins
- Ipsilateral upper extremity phlebitis or cellulitis
- Paralysis or lymphedema that may impede venous return
- Presence of dialysis graft/fistula in ipsilateral arm
- Hypercoagulable state (relative)
- Considerations
  - PICC line placed under fluoroscopy by interventional radiology for patients with:
    - Restricted peripheral access
    - Upper extremity venous thrombosis
  - End-stage renal disease patients
    - Peripheral veins spared for future fistula needs
    - Instead insert right internal jugular line
  - For frequent but intermittent access:
    - Insert venous port instead.

COMPLICATIONS

- Thrombus formation
  - Intraluminal: Inside the catheter. Attempt to dissolve with a small dose of alteplase
  - Mural: Between the catheter and the vein wall. Remove PICC line
- Arrhythmia
  - Occurs when inserted too far, irritates heart
- Phlebitis: Remove PICC line
- Line infection: Cultures from line, remove.

BASIC EQUIPMENT

- PICC kit contains most items for insertion
  - Betadine, alcohol swabs, sterile drapes, syringe, needle, introducer, catheter with guidewire, scissors, needle-driver, 3-0 silk suture, suture wing, gauze pads, tape measure
- Also needed:
  - Sterile gloves, saline and absorbent pad
  - Biopatch
  - Heparinized saline to "lock" Arrow catheter with a nonpressurized hub

SITES

- Either vein empties into the subclavian vein, which will be the position of the tip of the PICC line.
    - Cephalic vein—lies superiorly on the arm
    - Basilic vein—travels along the base of the arm and joins the brachial vein
- Measure from planned insertion site along the vessel course to the superior vena cava (third intercostal space).

PREPARATION

- Position patient
    - Abduct and externally rotate arm with elbow extended
- Identify the vein to be used
    - Prepare the area that will be punctured with alcohol then betadine
- Don mask, cap, sterile gown and gloves
- Place the sterile drape and absorbent pad
- Prepare equipment and prime PICC line.

PROCEDURE STEPS

- Anesthetize skin around vein with lidocaine without epinephrine
- Puncture skin with the introducer (stylet and cannula), advance until flash of blood
- Remove the stylet and insert the PICC catheter through the cannula
- Pull back and peel away the cannula from the catheter
- Lock with heparinized saline if needed
- Secure the line
    - If external line shorter than 1–1.5 inches, can use the manufactured securement device from the PICC tray to stabilize the line
    - If external line longer, secure by suturing catheter "wings" to skin
- Place biopatch at the insertion site
- Place sterile occlusive dressing over site and external line
- Post-procedure concerns
    - There is a tendency to bleed from the insertion site due to the introducer size
        - Restrict arm movement for the first 2 hours to minimize bleeding
    - Apply a pressure bandage directly on top of the occlusive dressing to avoid frequent redressing in the first 24 hours
        - A new PICC line should be redressed after 24 hours and then weekly unless there is an visualized ooze from the site
- Verifying PICC line positioning
    - Verify correct positioning of tip of PICC line with X-ray prior to use of the PICC line

– Measure and record the external PICC line length at the time of insertion and with each use to evaluate if there has been migration/change in external length.

USE OF ULTRASOUND TO ASSIST

- Modified-Seldinger: Access proximal veins
  - Using ultrasound guidance, a peripheral vein is accessed with a needle or an IV cannula
  - Guidewire is threaded in several centimeters then the needle or cannula is removed
  - Cut the skin beside the guidewire, and insert introducer sheath with dilator over the wire
  - Remove guidewire and dilator, PICC line is advanced through the introducer sheath, then the introducer is peeled away.

REMOVAL

- Aseptic technique required
- Remove the PICC slowly to minimize venospasm
  - Heat application may also help prevent minimize venospasm
- Do not apply excess force as this may fracture the catheter
  - Measure to ensure the PICC line is intact
  - Collect catheter tip for pathology if desired.

SELF-ASSESSMENT QUIZ

1. Which of the following is not a use for a peripherally inserted central catheter?
   a. CVP monitoring
   b. TPN administration
   c. Long-term antibiotic administration
   d. Blood draws
2. How often is a PICC line dressing changed?
   a. Daily
   b. Weekly
   c. Monthly
   d. With every line access
3. What do you do if, when you are setting up your sterile drape, the sterile side touches the bed?
   a. Nothing
   b. Wipe it down with alcohol
   c. Throw it away and get a new drape
   d. Let the patient know their insertion is not sterile and continue
4. Which of the following is not a contraindication to a PICC line?
   a. Phlebitis
   b. Contralateral mastectomy
   c. Trauma
   d. Thrombosis
5. During removal of the catheter, what is the proper method?
   a. Pull as quickly as possible
   b. Pull firmly, quickly and steadily
   c. Apply strong pressure against any resistance
   d. Slowly withdraw and stop if you meet resistance

Answers

1. a   2. b   3. c   4. b   5. d

SUGGESTED READING

1. Chopra V, Anand S, Hickner A, et al. Risk of venous thromboembolism associated with peripherally inserted central catheters: a systematic review and meta-analysis. Lancet. 2013;382:311.
2. Geffers C, Meyer E. No reason to conclude that maximal sterile barrier precautions do not reduce catheter-related blood stream infections. Ann Surg. 2011;253:212.
3. Grove JR, Pevec WC. Venous thrombosis related to peripherally inserted central catheters. J Vasc Interv Radiol. 2000;11:837.
4. Kost SI. Ultrasound-assisted venous access. Textbook of Pediatric Emergency Procedures, 2nd edition. In: King, C, Henretig, FM (Eds), Lippincott Williams and Wilkins, Philadelphia; 2008. p. 1255.
5. Liem TK, Yanit KE, Moseley SE, et al. Peripherally inserted central catheter usage patterns and associated symptomatic upper extremity venous thrombosis. J Vasc Surg. 2012;55:761.
6. Saseedharan S, Bhargava S. Upper extremity deep vein thrombosis. Int J Crit Illn Inj Sci. 2012;2:21.
7. Trerotola SO, Stavropoulos SW, Mondschein JI, et al. Triple-lumen peripherally inserted central catheter in patients in the critical care unit: prospective evaluation. Radiology. 2010;256:312.

Venous Cutdown

Crawford S

OBJECTIVES

- List the indications for venous cutdown
- Describe the complications of venous cutdown
- Know the contraindications for venous cutdown
- Be able to perform venous cutdown while maintaining sterile procedure

INTRODUCTION/BACKGROUND

- Venous cutdown is a procedure in which venous access may be rapidly obtained by cutting through skin and soft tissues, exposing a peripheral vein for IV insertion
- This is an alternative to venipuncture in critically ill patients in need of vascular access and are difficult to access
    - List may include shock patients, small children, sclerosed veins of intravenous drug users or in end stage renal disease.

UNIVERSAL PRECAUTIONS

- Sterile gloves must be worn while performing a cutdown
- Evaluate the need for face and eye protection as well as a gown.

OBTAIN INFORMED CONSENT

- Introduce yourself to the patient
- Explain the procedure to the patient, as well as the risks and benefits
- Gain informed consent to continue.

INDICATIONS

- When percutaneous access cannot be attained.

CONTRAINDICATIONS

- Coagulopathy
- Ipsilateral extremity injuries
- Vein thrombosis
- Cellulitis of overlying skin.

COMPLICATIONS

- Infection: Use strict asepsis
- Thrombophlebitis: Use silastic cannula instead of polyethylene cannula. Dilute solutions known to cause phlebitis
- Arterial cannulation: Occurs in infants
- Failure to find the vein: Do not attempt cutdown after previous thrombophlebitis or vein stripping
- Bleeding: Apply pressure if needed.

BASIC EQUIPMENT

- 3 mL syringe and 25 gauge needle
- Lidocaine
- Sterile skin prep, drape and gloves
- Gauze pads, tape
- Scalpel, curved hemostat, scissors
- 3-0 Silk suture
- Plastic venous dilator
- Intravenous catheter and tubing.

SITES

- Saphenous vein in the ankle is preferred
- It is consistently located 1 cm anterior and 1 cm superior to the medial malleolus
- Femoral—saphenous can also be reached by femoral cutdown, but this site is much less frequently used.

PREPARATION

- Cleanse skin
- Drape the area
- Infiltrate skin around the vein with lidocaine using a 25 gauge needle.

PROCEDURE STEPS

- Incise the skin through all its layers transversely across the vein (2.5 cm long)

- Dissect and mobilize 2 cm of the saphenous vein from its nerve using the curved hemostats
- Pass 2 sections of suture under the vein
  - Distally and proximally, tying distal suture
- Make a small incision in the vein and insert the dilator then the IV cannula
- Tie the proximal suture to secure the catheter
- Suture cannula to the skin at the exit point
- Suture the wound closed
- Apply sterile dressing: Gauze with antibiotic ointment and occlusive dressing over the top
- Tape cannula if needed.

REMOVAL

- Remove the sutures that tie the catheter in place and remove the catheter
- There are few complications if the catheter is removed within 24 hours
- However, once the vein has been used for cutdown, it frequently can no longer be used in future cannulation attempts.

SELF-ASSESSMENT QUIZ

1. What is the purpose of a venous cutdown?
   a. To give fluids
   b. To administer medications
   c. To give TPN
   d. To obtain access in a patient in whom all other attempts have failed
2. When is a venous cutdown not indicated?
   a. Coagulopathy
   b. When any other access is attainable
   c. Ipsilateral extremity injuries or cellulitis
   d. Vein thrombosis
3. What is the location of the saphenous vein in comparison to the medial malleolus?
   a. 2.5 cm distal, 2.5 cm posterior   b. 2.5 cm proximal, 2.5 cm anterior
   c. 1 cm proximal, 1 cm anterior   d. 1 cm distal, 1 cm posterior
4. When a patient has had venous cutdown, what is a common complication?
   a. Infection   b. Irritation
   c. Edema   d. Lymphedema
5. Which of the following vascular accesses are more preferred than cutdown?
   a. Central line   b. Peripheral line
   c. Peripherally inserted central line   d. All of the above

Answers

1. d   2. b   3. c   4. a   5. d

SUGGESTED READING

1. American College of Surgeons. Advanced Trauma Life Support (Student Manual). American College of Surgeons. 1997.
2. Britt LD, Weireter LJ Jr, Riblet JL, et al. Priorities in the management of profound shock. Surg Clin North Am. 1996;76:645.
3. Iserson KV, Criss EA. Pediatric venous cutdowns: Utility in emergency situations. Pediatr Emerg Care. 1986;2:231.
4. Kanter RK, Zimmerman JJ, Strauss RH, Stoeckel KA. Pediatric emergency intravenous access. Evaluation of a protocol. Am J Dis Child. 1986;140:132.
5. Kleinman ME, Chameides L, Schexnayder SM, et al. Part 14: Pediatric advanced life support: 2010 American Heart Association Guidelines for Cardiopulmonary Resuscitation and Emergency Cardiovascular Care. Circulation. 2010;122:S876.
6. Posner MC, Moore EE. Distal greater saphenous vein cutdown—technique of choice for rapid volume resuscitation. J Emerg Med. 1985;3:395.
7. Ralston M. Pediatric Advanced Life Support Provider Manual, American Heart Association, Subcommittee on Pediatric Resuscitation, Dallas; 2006. p.163.
8. Rosetti, VA, Thompson, BM, Aprahamian, et al. Difficulty and delay in intravascular access in pediatric arrests. Ann Emerg Med. 1984;13:406.

Chest X-ray Evaluation

Laks S

OBJECTIVES

- Understand basic steps of chest X-ray image interpretation
- Develop a consistent and thorough technique for reading images
- Learn how the silhouette sign can help localize pathology

INTRODUCTION/BACKGROUND

- There is no perfect way to read an X-ray
- However, adopt one method and use that approach consistently
- Check general info, then A-H, with an extended checklist for lateral films:
  - A. Airway
  - B. Bones
  - C. Cardiac
  - D. Diaphragm
  - E. Effusion
  - F. Fields (lung fields)
  - G. Gastric air bubble
  - H. Hilum.

DIRECTION OF X-RAY

- PA is taken with patient standing and X-rays pointing at the patient's back
  - Preferred imaging method
- AP is taken with patient sitting/laying, with X-rays pointing at the chest
  - Shows magnification of the heart and widening of the mediastinum
- In a lateral film, the left chest is against the film cassette which diminishes magnification of the heart and left ribs.

PROCEDURE STEPS

- General information
  - Check patient details
    - First name, surname, date of birth
  - Check orientation, position and side
    - Left, right, erect, AP, PA, supine, prone
  - Check additional information
    - Inspiration, expiration
  - Check adequacy of inspiration
    - Nine pairs of ribs should be seen posteriorly to have adequate inspiration
  - Check for rotation
    - Measure the distance from the medial end of each clavicle to the spinous process of the vertebra at the same level, should be equal
  - Check penetration
    - Should barely see the thoracic vertebrae behind the heart
  - Check exposure
    - Need to be able to identify both costophrenic angles and lung apices.
- A—Airway
  - Ensure trachea is visible and in midline
    - Trachea gets pushed away from abnormality, e.g. pleural effusion or tension pneumothorax
    - Or towards abnormality, e.g. atelectasis
    - Trachea normally narrows at the vocal cords
    - Carina angle between 60–100 degrees. Increase of this angle: Left atria enlargement, lymph node enlargement and left upper lobe atelectasis
    - Follow out both main stem bronchi
    - Check for tubes, pacemaker, wires, lines, foreign bodies, etc.
    - If ET tube is in place, the distal tip of the tube should be 3–4 cm above the carina
  - Check for a widened mediastinum
    - Mass lesions (e.g. tumor, lymph nodes)
    - Inflammation (e.g. mediastinitis, granulomatous inflammation)
    - Trauma and dissection (e.g. hematoma, aneurysm of the major mediastinal vessels).
- B—Bones
  - Check for fractures, dislocation, subluxation, osteoblastic or osteolytic lesions in clavicles, ribs, thoracic spine and humerus including osteoarthritic changes
  - At this time also, check the soft tissues for subcutaneous air and foreign bodies

- Caution with nipple shadows
  - Compare sides, if "lesion" is on both sides, they are shadows.
- C—Cardiac
  - Check heart size and heart borders
    - Borders appropriate or blunted
    - Thin rim of air around the heart, think of pneumomediastinum
    - Heart width should be <1/2 of lung width
  - Check aorta, SVC, IVC, azygos vein
    - Widening, tortuosity, (aorta for calcification)
  - Check heart valves
    - Calcification, valve replacements.
- D—Diaphragm
  - Right hemidiaphragm
    - Should be higher than the left
    - If much higher, think of effusion, lobar collapse, diaphragmatic paralysis
    - If you cannot see parts of the diaphragm, consider infiltrate or effusion
  - If taken in erect or upright position you may see free air under the diaphragm, if intra-abdominal perforation is present.
- E—Effusion
  - Effusions
    - Look for blunting of the costophrenic angle
    - Identify the major fissures, if you can see them more obvious than usual, then this could mean that fluid is tracking along the fissure
  - Check out the pleura
    - Thickening, loculations, calcifications and pneumothorax.
- F—Fields (lung fields)
  - Check for infiltrates
    - Identify infiltrates by use of known radiologic phenomenon, e.g. loss of heart borders or of the contour of the diaphragm
    - Identify which lobe is affected, know the location of lung fields: the right middle lobe abuts the heart, but the right lower lobe does not
    - The lingula abuts the left side of the heart
  - Check for granulomas, tumor and pneumothorax
  - Identify the pattern of infiltration
    - Interstitial pattern (reticular) versus alveolar (patchy or nodular) pattern
    - Lobar collapse
    - Look for air bronchograms, tram tracking, nodules, Kerley B lines
    - Pay attention to the apices.

- G—Gastric air bubble
  - Check correct position
  - Beware of hiatus hernia
  - Look for free air
  - Look for bowel loops between diaphragm and liver.
- H—Hilum
  - Check the position and size bilaterally
  - Enlarged lymph nodes
  - Calcified nodules
  - Mass lesions
  - Pulmonary arteries: If greater than 1.5 cm, think about possible causes of enlargement.

EXTENDED CHECKLIST FOR LATERAL FILMS

- B—Bones
  - Check the vertebral bodies and the sternum for fractures or other osteolytic changes.
- C—Cardiac
  - Check for enlargement of the right ventricle and right atrium (retrosternal and retrocardiac spaces)
  - Trace the aorta.
- D—Diaphragm
  - Check for fluid tracking up, costophrenic blunting and the associated hemidiaphragm.
- E—Effusions
  - Check to see the fissures here as well—both major fissures and the right lung's horizontal minor fissure may be found in the lateral view.
- F—Fields
  - Thoracic vertebrae: When there is a sudden change in transparency, then this is likely to be caused by infiltrate
  - Try to find the infiltrate that you think you saw on the PA-film to verify existence and anatomical location
  - Pay special attention to the lower lung lobes.

SILHOUETTE SIGN

- Can localize abnormalities on a PA-film without need for a lateral view
  - The loss of clarity of a structure suggests an area of differing density creating shadowing, such as a consolidated lung
  - Borders, outlines, edges on plain X-rays depend on the presence of two adjacent areas of different density
  - Differing densities:
    - Air, fat, soft tissue, liquid, calcium and contrast.

LUNG COLLAPSE

- Usually due to proximal occlusion of a bronchus, causing a loss of aeration
  - The remaining air is gradually absorbed, and the lung loses volume
  - May see tracheal displacement or mediastinal shift towards the collapse
  - Further findings are elevation of the hemidiaphragm, reduced vessel count on the side of the collapse or displacement of the opposite lung across the midline
- Most common causes:
  - Mucous plugging
  - Fluid retention in major airways
  - Inhaled foreign body
  - Malposition of an endotracheal tube
  - Proximal stenosing by bronchogenic carcinoma.

SELF-ASSESSMENT QUIZ

1. Pneumonia causes volume loss or collapse of the affected lung parenchyma
   a. True
   b. False
2. Opacification of what part of the lung will silhouette the right atrium?
   a. Left lower lobe
   b. Superior segment left lower lobe
   c. Right middle lobe
   d. Lingula
3. Which is a quality of a technically adequate PA chest radiograph?
   a. Thoracic spine disc spaces should be clearly visible through the heart
   b. The osseous detail of the thoracic spine is always clearly visualized
   c. The clavicular heads should be equal distance from the spinous processes
   d. Bronchovascular structures cannot be visualized through the heart
4. What is the correct order to read a chest X-ray?

1.	Bones	2.	Cardiac
3.	Lung fields	4.	Diaphragm
5.	Effusion	6.	Gastric air bubble
7.	Airway	8.	Hilum

   a. 1-2-3-4-5-6-7-8
   b. 8-7-6-5-4-3-2-1
   c. 7-3-4-2-5-1-6-8
   d. 7-1-2-4-5-3-6-8
5. Which of the following statements about the lateral chest X-ray is true?
   a. The right ribs are further away from the cassette and magnified less than the left
   b. The left chest is against the film cassette which diminishes magnification of the heart and left ribs
   c. The left ribs are usually projected posterior to the right ribs
   d. None of the above is true

Answers

1. b   2. c   3. c   4. d   5. b

SUGGESTED READING

1. Felson WB. Localization of Intrathoracic Disease. In: Felson WB (Ed). Chest Roentgenology. Saunders Co, Philadelphia. 1973. p. 22-70.
2. Goodman LR, Felson B. Felson's Principles of Chest Roentgenology: A Programmed Text. New York: WB Saunders; 1999.
3. Gottlieb RH, Hollenberg GM, Fultz PJ, Rubens DJ. Radiologic consultation: effect on inpatient diagnostic imaging evaluation in a teaching hospital. Acad Radiol. 1997;4(3):217-21.
4. Grainger RG, Allison D, et al. Grainger and Allison's Diagnostic Radiology: A Textbook of Medical Imaging, 4th Ed. New York: Saunders. 2001.
5. Moller TB, Reif E. Pocket Atlas of Radiographic Anatomy, 2nd Ed. New York: Thieme; 1999.
6. Netter F. Atlas of human anatomy. Summit, NJ: Ciba Pharmaceutical Co; 1998.
7. Pare JP, Fraser RS. Roentgenologic Signs in the diagnosis of Chest disease. In: Fraser RS, Muller NL. Synopsis of Diseases of the Chest. Saunders Co: Philadelphia; 1983. p. 164-87.
8. Pernkopf E, Platzer W. Pernkopf anatomy: Atlas of topographical and applied human anatomy. Baltimore: Urban & Schwarzenberg; 1989.
9. Squire LF. and R.A. Novalline. Squire›s Fundamentals of Radiology, 5th Ed. Cambridge: Harvard University Press; 1997.

28

EKG Interpretation

Farrag S

OBJECTIVES

- Describe the characteristics of a normal EKG complex
- Identify the physiological characteristics of normal conduction
- Identify normal sinus rhythm
- Compare and contrast EKG rhythms using an 8-step approach

INTRODUCTION/BACKGROUND

- Establish a consistent approach to evaluating the electrocardiogram (EKG)
- On every patient that has an EKG, spend time practicing, making sure to evaluate each case using a consistent method
- Consistency in evaluation steps will increase interpretation accuracy
- An EKG is obtained by placing electrical leads on the patient's chest
  - The leads are used to look at the heart from many angles
  - The EKG machine does not look at all the leads at once
  - The leads are recorded on a rhythm strip from each lead's viewpoint
    - Anterior: V3, V4
    - Septal: V1, V2
    - Inferior: II, III, and aVF
    - Lateral: I, aVL, V5 and V6.

UNIVERSAL PRECAUTIONS

- Wear gloves during performance of EKG.

OBTAIN CONSENT

- Introduce yourself to the patient
- Explain the procedure to the patient

- Explain that the procedure does not cause pain, however, during an EKG the patient needs to stay still.

INDICATIONS

- Evaluation of patients with implanted defibrillators and pacemakers
- Detection of myocardial injury, ischemia, and the presence of prior infarction
- Evaluation of the cardiac rhythm
- Evaluation of syncope
- Evaluation of metabolic disorders, side effects of pharmacotherapy, and cardiomyopathy.

CONTRAINDICATIONS

- No absolute contraindications
- In case of adhesive sensitivities, there are hypoallergenic lead options.

COMPLICATIONS

- Safe, routine procedure without major risks or complications
- Occasionally patients may have an allergic reaction to the adhesive in the electrodes.

BASIC EQUIPMENT

- EKG machine
- Electrodes
- Sheet or blanket for privacy.

PREPARATION

- Enter key patient information into the EKG machine
- The patient will be positioned on their back on a table or bed
- Cover the patient with a sheet and uncover only the chest.

PROCEDURE

- Attach the electrode to the lead wires
- Place the electrodes on the patient in the correct positioning for the individual leads
- Advise the patient to lie still
- Push the start/acquire button on the EKG machine
- Remove the lead wires and skin electrodes.

EKG ANALYSIS

- Step 1: Rate
- Step 2: Is the rhythm regular?
- Step 3: P wave before every QRS?
- Step 4: Axis deviation
- Step 5: Intervals—widths
- Heights
    - Step 6: Hypertrophy—P and QRS heights
    - Step 7: Ischemia or infarction—ST height
    - Step 8: T wave height.

ANALYSIS DETAIL

- Rate = Rule of 300: Divide 300 by the number of big boxes between each QRS
    - Normal heart rate is 60–100 beats per minute
    - >100 = tachycardia
    - <60 = bradycardia
- Step 2: Is the rhythm regular?
    - Evaluated by measuring the R-R distance and verifying that those distances are the same for each heartbeat
    - Irregular rhythms have varying R-R distances. Examples can include
        - Atrial fibrillation
        - Atrial flutter
        - PACs, PVCs
        - AV nodal blocks with variable conduction
- Step 3: P wave before every QRS?
    - Sinus rhythm has a P before every QRS
    - The shape and size of P waves should be uniform and smooth (same morphology)
    - Lack of normal P waves may include:
        - Atrial fibrillation
        - Atrial flutter
        - Wandering pacemaker
        - Multifocal atrial tachycardia
- Step 4: Axis deviation
    - LAD: LVH, LBBB left axis deviation: Negative AVF, positive lead I
    - RAD: RVH, RBBB right axis deviation: Positive AVF, negative lead I
    - Rule out hemiblock: Blockage of one limb of left bundle branch
        - Anterior LBBB hemiblock: Left axis deviation
        - Posterior LBBB: Right axis deviation

- Step 5: Normal widths
  - P wave: normal is .12 (3 small boxes)
    - Always begin from the left of the complexes and move to the right
    - The first width in a complex is the P wave width
    - Look specifically in lead II
      - If the duration of the P wave is greater than 0.12 seconds (3 small boxes) left atrial enlargement (LAE) exists
  - PR-i – normal is 0.20 sec (less than one large box)
    - As you move across the complex, the next width is the PR interval
    - This segment encompasses the entire P wave from its beginning up until the first deflection of the QRS complex
    - Less than 0.2 seconds (1 large box) is considered normal in adults
      - If the PR segment is greater than 0.2 seconds, first degree AV block exists
  - QRS: Normal is 0.08–0.10 sec (1–2 small boxes)
    - The next width is the QRS complex
    - Less than 0.12 (3 small boxes)
      - If more than 3 boxes, bundle branch block (BBB) exists (partial or full) or the complex had a ventricular origin
      - RBBB: RSR' in V1, 2 or 3
      - LBBB: deep, wide Q/S wave in V5 or V6
    - R wave progression in V1 to V6
      - R becomes more positive
      - Normal around V3 or V4
      - R/S ratio becomes >1
      - Poor progression: Possible past anterior MI
    - Pathologic Q wave: Suggests previous MI
      - >0.04 s in width and >2 mm in amplitude in more than one lead
      - OR Q wave amplitude >25% of the following R wave
  - QT interval: Normal is 450 ms in men, 460 in women
    - The next is the QT interval
    - The corrected QT (QTc) should be less than 0.45 (male) or 0.46 (female)
      - Half the R-R interval if there is a normal heart rate
      - Long QTc can lead to torsades de pointes
    - Causes of prolongation include:
      - Drugs (Na channel blockers)
      - Electrolytes: Low Ca, low Mg, low K
      - Hypothermia
      - Acute MI

- Congenital
- Increased ICP
- Step 6: Hypertrophy
  - Hypertrophy can be visualized as increased wave height
    1. The first height is of the P wave
       - If the P in lead II is greater than 2.5 small boxes, right atrial enlargement is probable (can also be biphasic with a tall initial component)
       - If the P wave in V1 is negative or biphasic (second component larger), then LAE likely. To be significant the negative portion in V1 should be >1 box wide and down
    2. PR segment: The only classic PR segment abnormality is PR depression
       - This is most often seen in the setting of pericarditis. Since there are multiple stages of pericarditis, these depressions are not always seen when this disease is present
    3. QRS complex
       - Right ventricular hypertrophy
         □ R>S in V1, but R wave gets smaller from V1 – V6. S wave persists in V5 and V6. RAD with slightly widened QRS
       - Left ventricular hypertrophy
         □ May see LAD with slightly widened QRS
         □ Evaluate using either:
           ◆ Add the S wave height of V1 to the R height of V5. LVH if >35 mm OR positive deflection in I or aVL >11 mV
- Step 7: Ischemia or MI
  - Height of ST segment
    - Begins with the J-point (end of QRS), slowly rising to the peak of the T and followed by a descent to the baseline
  - ST changes usually indicates ischemia
    - Elevation = Acute infarction
    - Depression = Ischemia
  - Remote ischemia: Q waves
- Step 8: T wave
  - T wave inversion = Ischemia
    - Symmetrical (left and right are mirror images)
    - Usually occurs in the same leads that demonstrate signs of acute infarction (Q waves and ST elevation)
  - T wave can also show hyperkalemia
    - Peaked T wave looks sharp enough to cut a finger

EKG INTERPRETATION

- There are many variations of the way that different rhythms may present
- Anything outside of the normal range is analyzed along with the patient's symptoms to create a working diagnosis
- However, there are several types of common abnormalities
- Sinus rhythm
  - Originating from SA node
  - Each P wave has the same morphology
  - P wave before every QRS
  - P wave in same direction as QRS
- Abnormal rate: Tachycardia
  - Regular rate with narrow complex: Sinus tachycardia, supraventricular tachycardia, atrial flutter
  - Regular rate with wide complex: Sinus tachycardia with aberrancy, supraventricular tachycardia with aberrancy, ventricular tachycardia
  - Irregular rate with narrow complex: Atrial fibrillation, atrial flutter with variable conduction, multifocal atrial tachycardia
  - Irregular rate with wide complex: Atrial fibrillation with aberrancy, atrial fibrillation with Wolff-Parkinson-White, ventricular tachycardia
- Abnormal PR-interval
  - First degree AV block
    - PR-interval is fixed and longer than 0.2 sec
  - Second degree block type 1-Wenckebach
    - PR-interval lengthens until a QRS drops
  - Second degree AV block Mobitz type 2
    - QRS drops randomly without PR lengthening
  - 3rd degree heart block (complete)
    - P wave has no relationship to the QRS
  - Sinus pause: SA node that misses a beat
- Ischemia location
  - Anterior (Anterior descending artery)
    - Q's in V1, V2, V3, and V4
  - Lateral (Circumflex coronary artery)
    - Q's in lateral leads I and AVL
  - Posterior (Right coronary artery)
    - Large R with ST depression in V1 and V2
  - Inferior (Right or left coronary artery)
    - Q's in inferior leads II, III, and AVF (diaphragmatic)

- Atrial flutter
  - Sharp, saw-tooth wave preceding the QRS instead of a P-wave (F-waves)
    - Step 1: Rate: 60-150
    - Step 2: Regular rhythm
    - Step 3: Several F-waves precede QRS
    - Step 4: Narrow complex (QRS duration 0.12)
    - Step 5: All complexes look the same
- Atrial fibrillation
  - A complete lack of P waves, and in their place a squiggly line, combined with an irregular heartbeat
- Each small box on the EKG strip represents 0.04 seconds on the horizontal axis.

SELF-ASSESSMENT QUIZ

1. The hallmark of atrial fibrillation is:
   a. Regular rhythm
   b. Fast pulse
   c. Irregular rhythm
   d. Slow pulse

2. A normal PR-interval is:
   a. 0.02 seconds
   b. 0.18 seconds
   c. 0.22 seconds
   d. 6 seconds

3. In sinus tachycardia, which of the following variables is abnormal?
   a. Rhythm
   b. Shape of complex
   c. PR interval
   d. Rate

4. A first-degree heart block may result in:
   a. Long QRS duration
   b. Fast rate
   c. Missed beats
   d. Long PR interval

5. The PR-interval is measured:
   a. From the beginning of the QRS to the end of the T-wave
   b. From the beginning to the end of the P-wave
   c. From the beginning of the P-wave to the beginning of the QRS
   d. From the end of the P-wave to the beginning of the QRS

Answers

1. c   2. b   3. d   4. d   5. c

SUGGESTED READING

1. Berger JS, Eisen L, Nozad V, et al. Competency in electrocardiogram interpretation among internal medicine and emergency medicine residents. Am J Med. 2005;118:873.
2. Fisch C, Ryan TJ, Williams SV, et al. Clinical competence in electrocardiography. Circulation. 1995;91:2683.
3. Fisch C. Evolution of the clinical electrocardiogram. J Am Coll Cardiol. 1989;14:1127.
4. Gillespie ND, Brett CT, Morrison WG, et al. Interpretation of the emergency electrocardiogram by junior hospital doctors. J Accid Emerg Med. 1996;13:395.
5. Hatala R, Norman GR, Brooks LR. Impact of a clinical scenario on accuracy of electrocardiogram interpretation. J Gen Intern Med. 1999;14:126.
6. Hevia AC, Fernández MM, Palacio JM, et al. EKG as a part of the preparticipation screening programme: An old and still present international dilemma. Br J Sports Med. 2011;45:776-9.
7. Hurst JW. The interpretation of electrocardiograms: Pretense or well-developed skill? Cardiol Clin. 2006;24:305.
8. Kadish AH, Buxton AE, Kennedy HL, et al. ACC/AHA clinical competence statement on electrocardiography and ambulatory electrocardiography. Circulation. 2001;104:3169.
9. Salerno SM, Alguire PC, Waxman HS. Competency in interpretation of 12-lead electrocardiograms: Recommendations from the American College of Physicians. Ann Intern Med. 2003;138:747.
10. Trzeciak S, Erickson T, Bunney B, et al. Variation in patient management based on EKG interpretation by emergency medicine and internal medicine residents. Am J Emerg Med. 2002;20:188.
11. Uberoi A, Stein R, Perez MV, et al. Interpretation of the electrocardiogram of young athletes. Circulation. 2011;124:746-57.
12. Vergara C. EKG rhythm interpretation patterns of medical interns: A needs assessment test. Conn Med. 2003;67(2):79-84.
13. Wisten A, Messner T. Symptoms preceding sudden cardiac death in the young are common but often misinterpreted. Scand Cardiovasc J. 2005;39:143-9.

Fluorescein Eye Examination

Maldonado MF

OBJECTIVES

- Describe the fluorescein staining technique and eye examination
- List the indications of fluorescein eye examination
- Know how to perform fluorescein eye examination

INTRODUCTION/BACKGROUND

- Fluorescein staining is used to confirm the diagnosis of corneal abrasion
  - Defects in epithelium appear green under blue light or a Wood's lamp
- Symptoms of corneal abrasion include eye pain and a foreign body sensation
  - Prior to the exam check: Visual acuity, penlight exam for signs of penetrating trauma, and eyelid inversion looking for foreign body.

UNIVERSAL PRECAUTIONS

- Gloves must be worn while performing eye examinations
- Evaluate the need for face and eye protection as well as a gown.

OBTAIN INFORMED CONSENT

- Introduce yourself to the patient
- Explain the procedure to the patient, as well as the risks and benefits
- Gain informed consent to continue.

INDICATIONS

- Patient with symptoms of corneal abrasion
  - Severe eye pain
  - Photophobia
  - Foreign body sensation.

CONTRAINDICATIONS

- Penetrating trauma
- Foreign body
- Nonreactive or irregular pupil
- Corneal infiltration or opacity
- Hypopyon
- Hyphema
- Angle closure glaucoma.

COMPLICATIONS

- Remove contacts prior to exam as fluorescein will permanently stain them.

BASIC EQUIPMENT

- Fluorescein strip
- 2 × 2 gauze
- Eye rinse solution
- Wood lamp.

SITES/POSITIONING

- The patient should be positioned for comfort, sitting upright with head tilted towards side of injury.

PREPARATION

- Procedure is performed in a completely dark environment, so turn off all light sources
- Have patient hold folded gauze under affected eye.

PROCEDURE STEPS

- Pull down lower lid, holding open the eye
- Moisten fluorescein strip with eye drop and allow the drop to run off the strip into the inferior cul-de-sac, or place the strip against the conjunctiva below the cornea. Inform the patient that fluorescein is a dark orange dye and have the patient blink 4–5 times, distributing the dye
- Visualize the cornea with a Wood's lamp
- Under Wood's lamp, corneal defects will appear green
    - Foreign bodies in the cornea may not stain, although the exposed edge of epithelium surrounding the foreign body will
    - A foreign body under an eyelid may cause corneal abrasions that appear as multiple linear abrasions in the same area, going in the same direction
    - Branching pattern of stain suggest herpes simplex infection
    - Contact lens abrasions are often central and round.

SELF-ASSESSMENT QUIZ

1. What are the indications for fluorescein eye exam?
   - a. Severe eye pain
   - b. Photophobia
   - c. Foreign body sensation
   - d. All of the above
2. Using Wood's lamp following fluorescein eye stain test exam, what color will a corneal abrasion be?
   - a. Blue
   - b. Green
   - c. Orange
   - d. Yellow
3. What should be checked prior to using fluorescein stain?
   - a. Eyelid inversion for foreign body
   - b. Visual acuity
   - c. Penlight exam for signs of penetrating trauma
   - d. All of the above
4. Which one of the following is not a sign of a possible foreign body?
   - a. There may be not stain
   - b. Just a small edge of epithelium may stain
   - c. Branching pattern of stain
   - d. There may be multiple linear abrasions in the same direction
5. Which of the following are contraindications to fluorescein stain?
   - a. Nonpenetrating trauma
   - b. Regular pupil
   - c. Corneal infiltration
   - d. Scleral injection

Answers

1. d   2. b   3. d   4. c   5. c

SUGGESTED READING

1. Dargin JM, Lowenstein RA. The painful eye. Emerg Med Clin North Am. 2008;26(1):199-216, viii.
2. Fraser S. Corneal abrasion. Clin Ophthalmol. 2010;4:387-90.
3. Schein OD. Contact lens abrasions and the nonophthalmologist. Am J Emerg Med. 1993;11(6):606-8.
4. Shields T, Sloane PD. A comparison of eye problems in primary care and ophthalmology practices. Fam Med. 1991;23:544.
5. Thyagarajan SK, Sharma V, Austin S, Lasoye T, Hunter P. An audit of corneal abrasion management following the introduction of local guidelines in an accident and emergency department. Emerg Med J. 2006;23(7):526-9.
6. Wilson SA, Last A. Management of corneal abrasions. Am Fam Physician. 2004;70(1):123-8.

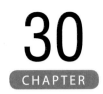

Conscious Sedation

Villa-Royval S

INTRODUCTION/BACKGROUND

- Conscious sedation is an altered state of consciousness that minimizes discomfort and anxiety using analgesics and sedatives
  - Patients are still able to speak and respond
  - Respiratory and cardiovascular functions remain adequate
  - Monitor heart rate, blood pressure, breathing, oxygen saturations, and alertness
  - Patients may have amnesia for the procedure.

UNIVERSAL PRECAUTIONS

- Gloves must be worn anytime as there may be a contact with bodily fluid.

OBTAIN INFORMED CONSENT

- Introduce yourself to the patient
- Explain the procedure to the patient, as well as the need for sedation
- Explain the major steps of sedation, as well as the risks and benefits
  - Risks: Pain, nausea, dizziness
  - Benefits: Improved comfort, relaxation, relief of pain
- Gain informed consent to continue.

INDICATIONS

- For painful or uncomfortable procedures
  - Like wound debridement, abscess drainage, reduction of fractures or dislocations, placement of central lines or chest tubes, endoscopy, colonoscopy
- Patients suitable for conscious sedation
  - Healthy
  - Mild systemic disease like hypertension
  - Severe nondecompensated systemic disease.

CONTRAINDICATIONS

- Severe decompensated systemic disease
- Patient for whom survival of the procedure is unlikely
- Lack of monitoring equipment or staff
- Recent ingestion of food or fluid.

COMPLICATIONS

- Inadequate amnesia or analgesia
- Hypoxia
- Hypoventilation
- Prolonged recovery.

BASIC EQUIPMENT

- IV access and medications
- Monitoring equipment
  - BP cuff, pulse oximeter, cardiac monitor
- Oxygen, nasal cannula or mask
- Resuscitation equipment
  - Endotracheal tubes, bag-valve mask, defibrillator, emergency cardiac drugs
- Reversal medication
  - Naloxone, flumazenil.

OPTIMAL SEDATION

- Patient is conscious and has purposeful response to commands
- Maintains airway, swallow and gag reflexes, spontaneous ventilations
- Is not anxious or afraid, is cooperative
- Experiences acceptable pain control and has mild amnesia for the procedure
- Has a minimal change in vital signs
- Recovers quickly to preprocedure status

OPIATE—ANALGESIC

- IV analgesic: Dose is titrated to effect
  - Morphine 0.1 mg/kg (2-4 mg) every 5 minutes, maximum dose 10-20 mg. Onset 2-3 minutes, peak 20 minutes, duration 2-4 hours
  - Fentanyl (for patients with morphine allergy) 25-50 µg IV every 6 minutes (maximum dose 250 µg). Onset 1-2 min, peak at 10-15 minutes. Duration 30-60 minutes.

BENZODIAZEPINES—SEDATIVES

- IV benzodiazepines are titrated to effect
  - Midazolam 0.5-1 mg every 2-3 minutes, maximum dose 0.2 mg/kg (or 5 mg). Onset in 1-3 min, peak in 5-7 min, duration 20-30 minutes
  - Lorazepam 1-2 mg every 3-4 min, maximum dose 4 mg. Onset 3-7 minutes, peak in 10-20 min, duration 6-8 hours
  - Diazepam 5 mg every 5 minutes to maximum dose of 20 mg. Onset 1-5 minutes, duration 1-8 hours.

PREPARATION

- Attach monitoring equipment
- Ensure patent IV line
- Obtain baseline vital signs
- Be aware that analgesics and sedatives may have synergistic effects
- Be aware that dosing must be adjusted for each patient based on their health, individual circumstances and age over 65 or under 18.

PROCEDURE STEPS

- Administer IV analgesics and sedatives
- Dose based on individual patient circumstances
- Do not begin procedure until adequate sedation has been achieved
- Begin off-titrating medication based on the length of the procedure
  - Reversal should not typically be needed if off-titrating is handled correctly.

MEDICATION REVERSAL

- Narcotic reversal: Naloxone
  - Competitive opioid receptor antagonist. Use 0.4 mg initially then 0.1-0.2 mg every 2-3 minutes as needed. May cause pulmonary edema, hypertension or increased sympathetic tone. Onset 1-2 minutes, peak effect 5 minutes. Duration of effect 30-45 minutes.
- Benzodiazepine reversal: Flumazenil
  - A pure antagonist. Give 0.2 mg IV over 15 seconds, may be give every minute as needed, (maximum 2-3 mg). Onset 1-2 minutes, peak 3 minutes, duration 10-15 minutes.

SELF-ASSESSMENT QUIZ

1. What is not true of conscious sedation?
   a. Patients are unable to speak and respond
   b. Respiratory functions remain adequate
   c. Cardiovascular functions remain adequate
   d. Patients may have amnesia for the procedure
2. Which is a benefit of conscious sedation?
   a. Pain   b. Nausea
   c. Relaxation   d. Dizziness
3. Flumazenil will antagonize the respiratory depression associated with which of the following medications?
   a. Morphine   b. Fentanyl
   c. Propofol   d. Lorazepam
4. What equipment should be in the room?
   a. Monitoring equipment   b. Resuscitation equipment
   c. Reversal medication   d. All of the above
5. Which medication has the longest duration?
   a. Midazolam   b. Lorazepam
   c. Diazepam   d. Flumazenil

Answers

1. a   2. c   3. d   4. d   5. b

SUGGESTED READING

1. American Society of Anesthesiologists Task Force on Sedation and Analgesia by Non-Anesthesiologists. Practice guidelines for sedation and analgesia by non-anesthesiologists. Anesthesiology. 2002; 96(4):1004-17.
2. Cohen LB, DeLegge MH, Aisenberg J, et al. AGA Institute Review of Endoscopic Sedation. Gastroenterology. 2007;133:675-701.
3. Horn E, Nesbit SA. Pharmacology and pharmacokinetics of sedatives and analgesics. Gastrointestinal Clinics of North America. 2004;14(2):247-68.
4. Lacy CF, Armstrong LL, Goldman MP, Lance LL. Drug Information Handbook. 11th Edition; Hudson, OH (Ed). American Pharmaceutical Association and Lexi-Comp Inc; 2003-2004.
5. McArdle P. Intravenous analgesia. Crit Care Clin. 1999;15(1):89-104.
6. McCaffery M, Pasero C. Pain: Clinical Manul. Phoenix, AZ: Mosby, Inc.1999; p. 382-5.
7. Ramsay MA, Savege TM, Simpson BR, Goodwin R. Controlled sedation with alphaxalone-alphadolone. Br Med J. 1974;2:656-9.
8. Rex DK. Moderate Sedation for Endoscopy: Sedation Regimens for Non-Anesthesiologists. Ailment Pharmacol Ther. 2006;24(2):163-71.
9. Volles D. University of Virginia Health System. Adult and Geriatric Sedation/Analgesia for Diagnostic and Therapeutic Procedures 2005. https://www.healthsystem.virginia.edu/internet/e-learning/drugchart_sedadult.pdf (Accessed November 14, 2014).

31

Primary Care Local and Regional Anesthesia (Local Infiltration, Field and Peripheral Nerve Block)

Villa-Royval S

OBJECTIVES

- Describe primary care local and regional anesthesia
- List the indications for local, field and peripheral nerve block
- Describe the complications of local and regional primary care anesthesia
- Be able to perform local and regional primary care anesthesia

INTRODUCTION/BACKGROUND

- Local anesthetic solution is infiltrated into the deep dermis within the procedural site
- The field block is applied subcutaneously surrounding the procedural area along its four borders
- Nerve block (regional) anesthetizes the nerve distribution distal to the injection.

UNIVERSAL PRECAUTIONS

- Sterile gloves should be worn while administering anesthetic
  - Many procedures that follow anesthesia should be performed with sterile technique.

OBTAIN INFORMED CONSENT

- Introduce yourself to the patient
- Explain the procedure to the patient, as well as the risks and benefits
- Gain informed consent to continue.

INDICATIONS

- Local anesthetic solution is used with small repairs or procedures
- The field block is used for larger areas, lasts longer than local and does not swell the procedural area
- Regional anesthesia (nerve block) is used when larger areas must be anesthetized, when local infiltration or field block would require large doses of anesthetic.

CONTRAINDICATIONS

- Allergy to anesthetic agent
- Infection at injection site
- Poor patient acceptance or cooperation
- Coagulopathy.

COMPLICATIONS

- Local toxicity
  - Prevent by using smallest effective dose
- Systemic toxicity
  - Use smallest effective dose
  - Aspirate prior to injection to ensure injection is not intravascular.

BASIC EQUIPMENT

- 10 mL syringe
- 18 gauge, 22–25 gauge needles
- Topical antiseptic
- Preferred anesthetic solution
- Sterile gloves
- Sterile drape.

TYPES OF ANESTHETICS

Agent	Class	Drug %	Onset	Duration	Max dose
Lydocaine (Xylocaine)	Amide	1	Rapid	30–60 min	4 mg/kg
Mepivacaine (Carbocaine)	Amide	1	Moderate	45–90 min	4 mg/kg
Bupivacaine (Marcaine)	Amide	0.25	Slow	2–4 hours	3 mg/kg
Procaine (Novocain)	Ester	1.0 to 2.0	Slow	15–60 min	7 mg/kg

(*Source:* Murphy MF. Local anesthetic agents. Emerg Med Clin North Am 1988; 6:769-76. Philip BK, Covino BG. Local and regional anesthesia. In: Wetchler BV, ed. Anesthesia for ambulatory surgery, 2d ed. Philadelphia: Lippincott, 1991:309-74.)

- Lidocaine is the most commonly chosen anesthetic due to rapid onset of action

EPINEPHRINE

- Epinephrine 1:100,000–1:200,000 dilution may be added to cause vasoconstriction, which decreases systemic absorption and prolongs the duration of anesthesia
  - Not used in nerve blocks as many nerves run adjacent to arterial vessels and intravascular injection could cause ischemia
  - Avoid causing vasoconstriction of the terminal arterial branches in the digits, tip of the nose, ear lobes, or tip of the penis.

PREPARATION

- Draw the anesthetic solution into a syringe with a large-bore needle (18 gauge)
- Place 22–25 gauge needle on anesthetic syringe in preparation for injection
- Sterile preparation of the area to be anesthetized with antiseptic solution and drape
- Stretching the skin at the injection site prior to injection may decrease discomfort.

PROCEDURE STEPS

- Local infiltration
  - Common anesthetic is 1–2% lidocaine
  - Puncture edge and advance into the procedural site
  - Aspirate to ensure needle is not intravascular
  - Inject anesthetic inside area, partially withdraw needle, redirect to ensure entire procedural tract is infiltrated
- Field block
  - Common anesthetic is 1–2% lidocaine
  - Puncture skin superior to site and advance subcutaneously along border
  - Aspirate to ensure needle is not intravascular
  - Inject anesthetic along one superior border, partially withdraw needle, redirect needle to apply anesthetic along second superior border
  - Remove needle, and repeat injection steps inferiorly, and redirect needle to anesthetize 2 inferior borders
- Nerve block
  - Anesthetic concentration limited to 1%
  - Inject into the extraneural or paraneural spaces
  - Blunt bevel needles may minimize nerve trauma
  - Always aspirate prior to injection
  - Site of injection depends upon area requiring anesthesia. Provider must be familiar with anatomy for proper procedure

Region	Nerves
Digit block	Anesthetize nerve on each side of digit
Wrist block	Anesthetize median, ulnar, radial and dorsal cutaneous nerve
Forehead	Supraorbital and supratrochlear nerve
Central face	Infraorbital nerve block
Ear	Supplied by multiple nerves and requires a field block
Dorsal foot	Saphenous, superficial and deep peroneal nerves
Plantar foot	Sural and posterior tibial nerves
Paracervical	Inject around cervix at 3, 6, 9 and 12 o'clock positions
Dorsal penile	Inject at 2 and 10 o'clock positions

SELF-ASSESSMENT QUIZ

1. Which of the following is true of a nerve block?
   a. Inject the inferior border
   b. Inject the superior border
   c. Inject anesthetic at the nerve distal to the wound
   d. Inject anesthetic at the nerve proximal to the wound
2. Which is the proper nerve to inject in a nerve wrist block?
   a. Median   b. Ulnar
   c. Radial   d. Dorsal cutaneous
   e. All of the above
3. Which of the following statements is true?
   a. In a nerve block, 2% anesthetic may be used
   b. Administer anesthesia with an 18 gauge needle
   c. 1–2% lidocaine is a common concentration for use in local infiltration
   d. Aspiration is never suggested prior to administering anesthetic
4. Which of the following statements is false regarding epinephrine?
   a. Causes vasodilation   b. Decreases systemic absorption
   c. Prolongs the duration of anesthesia d. Not used with nerve blocks
5. What is a potential complication of using epinephrine in anesthetic?
   a. Decreased systemic absorption
   b. Prolonged duration of anesthesia
   c. Ischemia in intravascular injection
   d. Ischemia in local infiltration of the skin of the trunk

Answers

1. d   2. e   3. c   4. a   5. c

SUGGESTED READING

1. Avina R. Primary care local and regional anesthesia in the management of trauma. Clin Fam Pract. 2000;2:533-50.
2. De Jong RH. Local anesthetics. St. Louis: Mosby; 1994. p. 345-80.
3. Glenn DM, Angel JM. Peripheral nerve blocks. In: Duke J, Rosenberg SG (Eds). Anesthesia secrets. Philadelphia: Hanley & Belfus; St. Louis: Mosby; 1996. p. 441-8.
4. Labat G, Adriani J. Labat's Regional anesthesia: Techniques and clinical applications, 4th ed. St. Louis: WH Green, 1985;107-30:193-235.
5. Murphy MF. Local anesthetic agents. Emerg Med Clin North Am. 1988;6:769-76.
6. Murphy MF. Regional anesthesia in the emergency department. Emerg Med Clin North Am. 1988;6:783-810.
7. Philip BK, Covino BG. Local and regional anesthesia. In: Wetchler BV (Ed). Anesthesia for ambulatory surgery, 2d ed. Philadelphia: Lippincott; 1991. p. 309-74.
8. Smith DW, Peterson MR, DeBerard SC. Regional anesthesia. Nerve blocks of the extremities and face. Postgrad Med. 1999;106:69-73,77-8.
9. Tetzlaff JE. The pharmacology of local anesthetics. Anesthesiol Clin North Am 2000;18:217-33.
10. Wedel DJ. Nerve blocks. In: Miller RD, Cucchiara RF (Eds). Anesthesia, 5th ed. Philadelphia: Churchill Livingstone; 2000. p. 1520-48.

Soft Tissue
Corticosteroid Injections

Vazquez G

INTRODUCTION/BACKGROUND

- Soft tissue corticosteroid injections can relieve inflammation; increase mobility, decrease swelling, heat and pain
    - Any acute or traumatic injury must be evaluated for appropriateness of injection
- Patients may respond to the first injection
    - Limit to no more than 4 injections per year
    - If 2 steroid injections fail to relieve symptoms, do not attempt further injections.

UNIVERSAL PRECAUTIONS

- Sterile gloves should be worn while performing soft tissue injection

OBTAIN INFORMED CONSENT

- Introduce yourself to the patient
- Explain the procedure to the patient, as well as the risks and benefits
- Gain informed consent to continue.

INDICATIONS

- Decreased mobility or pain
    - Bursitis
    - Trigger points

- Ganglion cysts
- Tenosynovitis
- Epicondylitis
- Carpal tunnel syndrome.

CONTRAINDICATIONS

- Local cellulitis
- Bacteremia
- Fracture
- Tendinopathies
- Relative contraindications
  - Minimal relief with prior injections
  - Uncontrolled diabetes mellitus
  - Uncontrolled coagulopathy or anticoagulation
  - Osteoporosis.

COMPLICATIONS

- Infection—use sterile procedure
- Systemic reaction
  - Alterations in taste or hyperglycemia
- Local reaction to medication
  - Allergic: Swelling, tenderness, warmth
  - Fat atrophy
  - Local depigmentation
- Injury to surrounding structures
  - Nerves, tendons (be aware of anatomy).

BASIC EQUIPMENT

- Sterile and nonsterile gloves
- Sterile drapes, skin prep solution
- 4 × 4 sterile gauze
- Anesthetic
- Corticosteroid
- 1–10 mL syringes
- Needles, 18 gauge and 22–25 gauge
- Bandage.

MEDICATION FOR INJECTION

- Corticosteroid—provides long-term symptom relief
  - Triamcinolone
  - Methylprednisolone

- Hydrocortisone
- Betamethasone
- Anesthetic - dilutes concentrated steroid, provides quick, short-lasting pain relief
  - Lidocaine or bupiviacaine.

PREPARATION

- Identify the needle insertion site
- Prepare the skin with antiseptic solution and drape
- Apply ice or topical cooling spray to provide temporary cutaneous analgesia.

PROCEDURE STEPS

- Insert the needle through the skin to the depth of the desired injection
  - Aspirate to confirm needle not intravascular
- Slowly inject. If resistance is met, the needle tip may be against bone, may reposition by withdrawing slightly
- Remove needle and place bandage on site
- Instruct patient to rest the area for 2 days to minimize post-injection injury.

SELF-ASSESSMENT QUIZ

1. Which of the following is a systemic reaction that could occur following soft tissue corticosteroid injection?
   a. Hyperglycemia
   b. Swelling
   c. Tenderness
   d. Warmth
2. Which of the following provide quick pain relief?
   a. Methylprednisolone
   b. Hydrocortisone
   c. Betamethasone
   d. Lidocaine
3. Which of the following is not an indication for injection?
   a. Bursitis
   b. Fracture
   c. Ganglion cysts
   d. Tenosynovitis
4. Which of the following is a contraindication for soft tissue corticosteroid injection?
   a. Local cellulitis
   b. Bacteremia
   c. Tendinopathies
   d. All of the above
5. How often can a soft tissue corticosteroid injection be repeated?
   a. Once a week
   b. Once a month
   c. Once every 3 months
   d. Once a year

Answers

1. a   2. d   3. b   4. d   5. c

SUGGESTED READING

1. Assendelft WJ, Hay EM, Adshead R, Bouter LM. Corticosteroid injections for lateral epicondylitis: A systematic overview. Br J Gen Pract. 1996;46:209-16.

2. Bisset L, Beller E, Jull G, Brooks P, Darnell R, Vicenzino B. Mobilisation with movement and exercise, corticosteroid injection, or wait and see for tennis elbow: Randomised trial. BMJ. 2006;333(7575):939.

3. Foley B, Christopher TA. Injection therapy of bursitis and tendinitis. In: Roberts JR, Hedges JR, Chanmugan AS (Eds): Clinical Procedures in Emergency Medicine. 4th ed. Philadelphia, Pa.: WB Saunders; 2004. p. 1020-40.

4. Hay EM, et al. A pragmatic randomised controlled trial of local corticosteroid injection and physiotherapy for the treatment of new episodes of unilateral shoulder pain in primary care. Ann Rheum Dis. 2003;62(5):394-99.

5. Nelson KH, Briner W Jr, Cummins J. Corticosteroid injection therapy for overuse injuries. Am Fam Physician. 1995;52:1811-6.

6. Owen DS. Aspiration and injection of joints and soft tissues. In: Kelley WN (Ed). Textbook of rheumatology. 5th ed. Philadelphia: Saunders. 1997:591-608.

7. Pfenninger JL. Joint and soft tissue aspiration and injection. In: Pfenninger JL, Fowler GC, (Eds). Procedures for primary care physicians. St. Louis: Mosby; 1994. p.1036-54.

8. Wang AA, Hutchinson DT. The effect of corticosteroid injection for trigger finger on blood glucose level in diabetic patients. J Hand Surg. 2006;31(6):979-81.

Splinting

Vazquez G

INTRODUCTION/BACKGROUND

- Splinting immobilizes injured extremities to prevent further injury, decrease pain and allow for healing
  - After reduction of a dislocated joint, splints maintain proper positioning
  - Stabilizing a fracture with a splint keeps bones in their proper alignment
  - Patients with strained ligaments have their extremity splinted in the position of function to decrease pain.

UNIVERSAL PRECAUTIONS

- Gloves must be worn while using splinting materials and when open wounds are present
- Evaluate the need for face and eye protection as well as a gown.

OBTAIN INFORMED CONSENT

- Introduce yourself to the patient.
- Explain the procedure to the patient, as well as the risks and benefits
- Instruct patients that after the splint is applied, if there is worsening pain, swelling, discoloration, difficulty moving fingers or toes or change in sensation to return
- Gain informed consent to continue.

INDICATIONS

- Fracture
- Dislocation
- Sprain
- Tendon lacerations.

CONTRAINDICATIONS

- No absolute contraindication
- Consider prior to placing a splint
  - Likelihood for severe swelling as even splints can become restrictive with severe swelling
  - If neurovascular compromise is present prior to splinting, attempt reduction prior to placing a splint.

COMPLICATIONS

- Neurovascular compromise
- Compartment syndrome
- Pressure sore
- Burn.

BASIC EQUIPMENT

- Stockinette
- Cotton padding
- Plaster or fiberglass rolls
- Elastic bandages with clips or tape
- Heavy duty scissors
- Water
- Sheet.

SITES/POSITIONING

- Expose the injury site fully prior to splinting. All injuries to the extremity must be identified prior to splinting
- Evaluate pulses, motor and sensory function prior to splinting
- Treat skin or soft tissue injuries prior to splinting.

PREPARATION

- Drape the patient with a sheet to protect clothing prior to splinting
- Remove all jewelry from the extremity
- Administer analgesics or anesthetics prior to splinting or reductions
- Reduce fractures or dislocations prior to splinting
- Position patient to give you access to the extremity but also be comfortable

PROCEDURE STEPS

- Apply stockinette to extremity to protect skin to a length longer than splint length
- Place cotton padding material over stockinette for comfort and to allow for swelling, in two layers, overlapping the previous layer by 25–50% each roll
    - Wrap extremity in final desired position
- Measure plaster for length and lay out the correct length
    - 8 layers for arms and 12 layers for legs
- Immerse material in water until it is saturated, then remove excess of water from layers using pressure applied by a finger on each side squeezing water in a downward motion
- Place the plaster material over the cotton padding, molding it to the contours of the extremity
- Apply a cotton layer to hold the splint in place, then fold stockinette over edges
- Secure splint with an elastic bandage, wrapping distal to proximity without excessively compressing the extremity
- Ensure the extremity is in anatomical position and mold the splint if needed
    - Instruct patient to remain still as it dries
- Check neurovascular status, positioning, splint strength, patient comfort
- X-rays may be used to verify positioning.

REMOVAL

- Remove after swelling has had adequate time to resolve
- Unwrap elastic bandage, remove plaster sides and cut cotton and stockinette carefully off.

SELF-ASSESSMENT QUIZ

1. What is true regarding the purpose of splinting?
    - a. Prevents further injury
    - b. Decreases pain
    - c. Provides stability for healing
    - d. All of the above
2. What holds the plaster in place?
    - a. Tape
    - b. Cotton
    - c. Stockinette
    - d. Elastic bandage
3. Which types of injuries can a splint be used on?
    - a. Dislocations
    - b. Fractures
    - c. Sprains
    - d. All of the above
4. When should the splint be removed?
    - a. At 48 hours
    - b. At 72 hours
    - c. When swelling is resolved
    - d. When pain is resolved
5. What complication of splinting can have the worst effect on the extremity?
    - a. Compartment syndrome
    - b. Pressure sore
    - c. Burn
    - d. None of the above

Answers

1. d   2. b   3. d   4. c   5. a

SUGGESTED READING

1. Avina R. Primary care local and regional anesthesia in the management of trauma. Clin Fam Pract. 2000;2:533-50.
2. Glenn DM, Angel JM. Peripheral nerve blocks. In: Duke J, Rosenberg SG (Eds). Anesthesia secrets. Philadelphia: Hanley & Belfus; St. Louis: Mosby; 1996. p. 441-8.
3. Melone CP Jr, Isani A. Anesthesia for hand injuries. Emerg Med Clin North Am. 1985;3:235-43.
4. Nishanian E, Gargarian M. Regional anesthesia. In: Hurford WE (Ed). Clinical anesthesia procedures of the Massachusetts General Hospital, 5th ed. Philadelphia: Lippincott-Raven; 1998. p. 264-86.
5. Smith DW, Peterson MR, DeBerard SC. Regional anesthesia. Nerve blocks of the extremities and face. Postgrad Med. 1999;106:69-73,77-8.
6. Tetzlaff JE. Peripheral nerve blocks. In: Morgan GE, Mikhail MS (Eds). Clinical anesthesiology, 2d ed. Stamford, Conn.: Appleton & Lange; 1996. p. 245-71.
7. Wedel DJ. Nerve blocks. In: Miller RD, Cucchiara RF. Anesthesia, 5th ed. Philadelphia: Churchill Livingstone, 2000:1520-48.
8. Zuber TJ. Skin biopsy, excision, and repair techniques. The illustrated manuals and videotapes of soft tissue surgery techniques. Kansas City: American Academy of Family Physicians; 1998.

Arthrocentesis

Gonzalez GA

INTRODUCTION/BACKGROUND

- Most joints can be punctured to remove synovial fluid
- The most common reason for aspiration is a red, painful, swollen joint with limited range of motion
  - Diagnostic to identify cause
  - Therapeutic drainage to relieve pain
  - Instillation of medication.

UNIVERSAL PRECAUTIONS

- Sterile gloves must be worn while performing joint aspiration
- Evaluate the need for face and eye protection as well as a gown.

OBTAIN INFORMED CONSENT

- Introduce yourself to the patient
- Explain the procedure to the patient, as well as the risks and benefits
- Gain informed consent to continue.

INDICATIONS

- Diagnostic arthrocentesis:
  - Evaluation of arthritis
  - Evaluation of joint effusion

- – Identification of intra-articular fracture
- – Identification of crystal arthropathy
- Therapeutic arthrocentesis:
  - – Relief of pain by aspirating effusion or blood
  - – Drainage of septic effusion
  - – Instillation of anti-inflammatory or anesthetic.

CONTRAINDICATIONS

- Overlying cellulitis—if joint was tapped through cellulitis admit for IV antibiotics, even if aspirate is not infectious
- Relative contraindications
  - – Skin lesion or dermatitis overlying the joint
  - – Known bacteremia
  - – Adjacent osteomyelitis
  - – Uncontrolled coagulopathy
  - – Bleeding diatheses
  - – Joint prosthesis—tapped by an orthopedist.

COMPLICATIONS

- Cartilage damage—prevent by not advancing the needle into the joint space once synovial fluid enters the syringe
- Bleeding—usually self corrects
- Infection—use sterile procedure.

BASIC EQUIPMENT

- Sterile gloves and drapes
- 4 × 4 sterile gauze
- Skin preparatory solution
- Lidocaine 1%
- Syringes
- Needles, 18 gauge and 25 or 27 gauge
- Hemostat
- Specimen tubes.

SITES/POSITIONING

- Knee—parapatellar preferred
- Hip aspiration—by specialists
- Shoulder anterior—medial to head of humerus, 1 cm lateral to coracoid
- Elbow—between lateral epicondyle of humerus and olecranon process of ulna

- Finger—dorsomedially or dorsolaterally
- Ankle—anteriomedial, between medial malleolus and extensor hallucis.

PREPARATION

- Identify the needle insertion site
- Prepare the skin with antiseptic solution and drape
- Use a 25 or 27 gauge needle to inject 2–5 mL of local anesthetic (lidocaine 1%) into the subcutaneous tissues.

PROCEDURE STEPS

- Insert the 18 gauge needle into the joint space while gently aspirating until synovial fluid enters the syringe
- If a bone is encountered during needle insertion, pull the needle back, verify the landmarks, and redirect the needle
- If fluid stops flowing into the syringe
  - Redirect needle and continue to aspirate
  - Apply gentle pressure around joint
- Remove needle and place bandage on site.

SELF-ASSESSMENT QUIZ

1. Which is a reason to aspirate a joint?
   - a. Diagnostic
   - b. Therapeutic drainage
   - c. Instillation of medication
   - d. All of the above
2. Which is not a physical sign commonly seen prior to tapping a joint?
   - a. Red joint
   - b. Full joint range of motion
   - c. Joint pain
   - d. Swollen joint
3. What should be done first if fluid stops flowing into the syringe?
   - a. Remove the needle
   - b. Apply joint pressure
   - c. Redirect needle
   - d. Advance the needle
4. What size needle should be used to aspirate the joint?
   - a. 23
   - b. 21
   - c. 18
   - d. 14
5. What is the correct joint and positioning combination?
   - a. Finger—dorsomedially
   - b. Knee—posterior fossa
   - c. Shoulder—lateral humeral head
   - d. Ankle—posterior, on either side of Achilles

Answers

1. d   2. b   3. c   4. c   5. a

SUGGESTED READING

1. Barry III J, Christian CL, Sculco TP. Manual of rheumatology and outpatient orthopedic disorders, diagnosis and therapy, 1st ed. Boston: Little, Brown & Co; 1981.
2. Margaretten ME, Kohlwes J, Moore D, Bent S. Does this adult patient have septic arthritis? JAMA 2007;297(13):1478-88.
3. Reichman EF and Simon RR. Emergency Medicine Procedures. 1st ed. New York: McGraw Hill; 2004.
4. Self WH, Wang EE, Vozenilek JA, del Castillo J, Pettineo C, Benedict L. Dynamic emergency medicine. Arthrocentesis. Acad Emerg Med. 2008;15(3):298.
5. Siva C, Velazquez C, Mody A, Brasington R. Diagnosing acute monoarthritis in adults: A practical approach for the family physician. Am Fam Physician. 2003;68(1):83-90.
6. Thomsen TW, Shen S, Shaffer RW, Setnik GS. Videos in clinical medicine. Arthrocentesis of the knee. N Engl J Med. 2006;354(19):e19.
7. Zhang Q, Zhang T, Lv H, Xie L, Wu W, Wu J, et al. Comparison of two positions of knee arthrocentesis: How to obtain complete drainage. Am J Phys Med Rehabil. 2012;91(7):611-5.
8. Zuber TJ. Knee joint aspiration and injection. Am Fam Physician. 2002;66(8):1497-500, 1503-4, 1507.

Closed Joint Reductions

Gonzalez GA

OBJECTIVES

- Describe close joint reduction technique
- List the indications for joint reduction
- Describe the complications
- Know how to perform shoulder, hip and ankle reductions

INTRODUCTION/BACKGROUND

- Reduction is repositioning a joint to its normal position after injury
  - To minimize soft tissue complications
  - Restore alignment, length, rotation
- Reduction maneuver is specific to joint
  - Muscles contract, holding joint out of the normal alignment
- Consider IV sedation prior to reduction.

UNIVERSAL PRECAUTIONS

- Gloves must be worn whenever there is a risk of bodily fluid contact
- Evaluate the need for face and eye protection as well as a gown.

OBTAIN INFORMED CONSENT

- Introduce yourself to the patient
- Explain the procedure to the patient, as well as the risks and benefits
- Gain informed consent to continue.

INDICATIONS

- Clinically or radiographically dislocated joint.

CONTRAINDICATIONS

- Shoulder: Humeral fracture
- Radial head: Radial fracture
- Ankle: Tibial fracture.

COMPLICATIONS

- Fracture—splint and consult orthopedics
- Failure to reduce—splint and immobilize, consult orthopedics
- Nerve or blood vessel damage
- Blood clots.

BASIC EQUIPMENT

- Ankle: Cast padding
  - Fiberglass
  - Lukewarm water
  - Ace bandages
  - Gloves
- Shoulder: Immobilizer
- Elbow: Sling.

PROCEDURES

- Elbow dislocation—Radius
  - Seat patient with injured hand in their lap
  - Provider takes injured hand in a handshake position, with the other hand behind the elbow, thumb on radial head
    - Pull longitudinal traction and supinate the forearm while keeping radial pressure with the thumb
  - Check post-reduction X-rays, place in splint
- Ankle dislocation
  - Seat patient with legs dangling
  - Assistant place pressure on patient's thighs
  - Grasp forefoot with one hand and heel with other, twist foot to the side of the dislocation
  - Apply longitudinal traction in the reverse direction of lateral force
  - Check post-reduction X-ray, splint foot
- Shoulder dislocation
  - Position patient supine with head of bed at 30 degrees and bed at provider's waist level. Patient's injured arm should be at the edge of the bed
    - Wrap sheet around patient's trunk
      - Tie to the bedrail on the uninjured side

    – Tie injured forearm with elbow at 90 degrees by sheet to providers waist
- Provider should lean back with arm abducted to 30 degrees and internally rotated 15–30 degrees

    – Hold traction for several minutes until the patient's shoulder muscles fatigue
- Posterior dislocation: Rotate arm internally
- Anterior dislocation: Externally rotate and abduct arm

    – May need to apply pressure on humeral head with provider's hand
    – Shoulder should click back into position.

SELF-ASSESSMENT QUIZ

1. Which of the following is not true about reduction?
   a. Reduction is repositioning a joint to its normal position after injury
   b. All reductions are performed in the same way
   c. Is performed to minimize soft tissue complications
   d. Reductions also restore alignment, length, rotation
2. When should a reduction be performed?
   a. When there is a limb length discrepancy
   b. When there is joint pain following an injury
   c. When there is evidence of dislocation on X-ray
   d. When there is a fracture on X-ray
3. What grip does the provider take when reducing an elbow dislocation?
   a. Hold humerus
   b. Hold forearm and humerus
   c. Handshake injured hand and pronate
   d. Handshake injured hand and supinate
4. What should not be done after reduction?
   a. Check position by X-ray
   b. Cast extremity
   c. Splint extremity
   d. Give pain medications
5. What is the most important step in any joint reduction?
   a. Applying an overwhelmingly strong force
   b. Applying a twisting pressure
   c. Applying a sustained pressure
   d. Applying pressure with a jerking motion

Answers

1. b   2. c   3. d   4. b   5. c

SUGGESTED READING

1. Bell S, Salmon J. The management of common dislocations in the upper limb. Aust Fam Physician. 1996;25(9):1413-5,1418-23.

2. Canale ST, James HB. Fractures and Dislocation, Part XV. Campbell's Operative Orthopaedics, 11th ed. Philadelphia: Mosby Elsevier; 2008.

3. Chapman MW. Chapman's Orthopaedic Surgery, 3rd ed. Philadelphia: Lippincott, Williams & Wilkins; 2001.

4. Eachempati KK, Dua A, Malhotra R, Bhan S, Bera JR. The external rotation method for reduction of acute anterior dislocations and fracture-dislocations of the shoulder. J Bone Joint Surg Am. 2004;86-A(11):2431-4.

5. Kuhn MA, Ross G. Acute elbow dislocations. Orthop Clin North Am. 2008;39(2):155-61.

6. Rivera F, Bertone C, De Martino M, Pietrobono D, Ghisellini F. Pure dislocation of the ankle: three case reports and literature review. Clin Orthop Relat Res. 2001. p. 179-84.

7. Robert JR, Hedges RJ. Clinical Procedures in Emergency Medicine. 4th ed. Philadelphia, PA: W.B. Saunders Company; 2004.

8. Westin CD, Gill EA, Noyes ME, Hubbard M. Anterior shoulder dislocation. A simple and rapid method for reduction. Am J Sports Med. 1995;23(3):369-71.

Fetal Heart Rate Monitoring

Kupesic Plavsic S

OBJECTIVES

- Know how to perform fetal heart rate monitoring
- Be able to interpret fetal heart rate monitoring

INTRODUCTION/BACKGROUND

- Electronic fetal monitoring is used to assess fetal wellbeing
- Interpreting the results of the fetal heart rate monitoring the same way every time increases the accuracy and consistency of interpretation
- Understand the features of reassuring fetal heart rate strips, and recognize the ones of concern and problematic ones that require intervention.

UNIVERSAL PRECAUTIONS

- Gloves must be worn if there is any contact with bodily fluids.

OBTAIN INFORMED CONSENT

- Introduce yourself to the patient
- Patients should be educated regarding fetal heart rate monitoring.

INDICATIONS

- Intermittent monitoring can be used with low-risk pregnancies
  - Record strips every half hour in the first stage of labor, every 15 minutes in the second stage
- Continuous monitoring is used with high-risk pregnancies
  - Review tracings every 15 minutes in the first stage, every 5 minutes in the second stage

CONTRAINDICATIONS

- None

COMPLICATIONS

• None

PREPARATION

• Obtain at minimum a 10-minute fetal heart rate strip.

PROCEDURE STEPS

- Determine baseline fetal heart rate (FHR) over 10 minutes (not during contractions). Normal baseline FHR is from 110 to 160 beats per minute (bpm)
- Bradycardia: Baseline FHR less than 110 bpm
- Tachycardia: Baseline FHR greater than 160 bpm
• Variability is the fluctuations of the baseline in a ten minute segment of tracing
- Absent: No fluctuations
- Minimal: Fluctuations less than 5 bpm
- Moderate (normal): Amplitude range 6–25 bpm
- Marked: Amplitude range greater than 25 bpm
• Number of contractions in 10 minutes
- Normal is less than 5 contractions in a 10-minute period
- Tachysystole is more than 5 contractions in a 10 minute period
• Periodic fetal heart rate changes are the accelerations or decelerations that occur in relation to contractions
- Accelerations are increases in heart rate: Peak within 30 seconds and return to baseline within 2 minutes
- Decelerations are decreases in heart rate.

ACCELERATIONS

• An abrupt increase in the FHR that is visually apparent. Peak must be at least 15 bpm above baseline, must be at least 15 seconds and less than two minutes
• Prolonged accelerations are at least 2 minutes long, but less than 10 minutes in duration

DECELERATIONS

• Are classified based upon their timing related to contractions
- Early decelerations have onset, peak and return to baseline at the same time as the contraction
- Late decelerations begin at the contraction peak and end after the contraction ends

– Variable decelerations may occur at any time in relation to the contraction
– Prolonged decelerations is a decrease from the baseline of at least 15 bpm that lasts at least 2,but less than 10 minutes.

TRACING CLASSIFICATION

- Category I is a normal tracing
  – Normal FHR, moderate variability, no late or variable decelerations
- Category II is an intermediate tracing
  – All strips not category I or III
- Category III are abnormal
  – Sinusoidal pattern (fixed periodicity) or
  – Absent baseline FHR variability with either: Recurrent late decelerations; recurrent variable decelerations; or bradycardia.

MANAGEMENT

- Category I: Normal, no fetal indications to change labor management
- Category II: Evaluate maternal vitals, cervical status, reposition the mother, administer maternal oxygen or IV fluids, stop oxytocin, consider amnioinfusion
- Category III: Consider immediate delivery.

SELF-ASSESSMENT QUIZ

1. A resident is caring for a patient in active phase of labor and notes a late deceleration of the monitor strip. The most appropriate action is to:
   a. Place the mother in supine position
   b. Administer oxygen via face mask
   c. Increase the rate of IV Pitocin
   d. Document the findings and continue to monitor FHR without notifying the attending

2. An intern is performing an assessment of a patient who is scheduled for C-section. Which of the findings require immediate consultation with the supervising physician?
   a. Maternal pulse rate of 80 bpm   b. White blood cell count of 9,000
   c. Fetal heart rate of 190 bpm   d. Hemoglobin of 12 g/dL

3. An intern is caring for a patient in labor who is on Pitocin infusion. Which of the findings would indicate that the Pitocin infusion needs to be discontinued?
   a. Two contractions occurring in a 10-minute period
   b. Three contractions occurring in a 10-minute period
   c. A fetal heart rate of 90 beats per minute
   d. A fetal heart rate of 120 beats per minute

Contd...

Contd...

4. A resident is caring for a patient in labor and is monitoring the fetal heart rate. Baseline FHR is from 140 to150 bpm. She notes the presence of an abrupt increase in the FHR of about 20–25 bpm above baseline lasting one minute. Which of the following actions is most appropriate?
   a. Notify the supervising physician of the findings
   b. Prepare the patient for C-section
   c. Reposition the mother and administer oxygen via mask
   d. Document the findings and inform the mother that FHR monitoring indicates fetal wellbeing

5. A resident monitoring a patient in labor notices minimal variability of fetal heart rate accompanied by decelerations occurring after the peak of each contraction. There are three contractions occurring in a 10 minute period. Amplitude range of FHR tracing is 2–3 beats per minute. Which of the following options most accurately defines the problem?
   a. Late decelerations and minimal variability are suggestive of placental insufficiency
   b. Early decelerations and moderate variability suggest normal FHR tracing
   c. Variable decelerations and minimal variability are suggestive of head compression
   d. Variable decelerations and moderate variability are suggestive of placental insufficiency

Answers

1. b   2. c   3. c   4. d   5. a

SUGGESTED READING

1. American College of Obstetricians and Gynecologists. ACOG Practice Bulletin. Clinical Management Guidelines for Obstetrician-Gynecologists. 2005; Number 70.
2. American College of Obstetricians and Gynecologists. ACOG Practice Bulletin No. 106: Intrapartum fetal heart rate monitoring: nomenclature, interpretation, and general management principles. Obstet Gynecol. 2009;114:192.
3. American College of Obstetricians and Gynecologists. Practice bulletin no. 116: Management of intrapartum fetal heart rate tracings. Obstet Gynecol. 2010;116:1232.
4. Bailey R. Intrapartum Fetal Monitoring. Am Fam Physician. 2009;80(12):1388-96.
5. Macones GA, Hankins GD, Spong CY, Hauth J, Moore T. The 2008 National Institute of Child Health and Human Development workshop report on electronic fetal monitoring: Update on definitions, interpretation, and research guidelines. Obstet Gynecol. 2008;112(3):661-6.
6. Montgomery L, Kupesic S, Molokwu J. Normal Pregnancy. In: Intern Tips in Obstetrics and Gynecology. New Delhi: Jaypee; 2014 (in press).
7. Parer JT, Ikeda T. A framework for standardized management of intrapartum fetal heart rate patterns. Am J Obstet Gynecol. 2007;197:26.e1.

37

Internal Fetal Heart Rate Monitoring

Mendez MD, Kupesic Plavsic S

OBJECTIVES

- List the indications for intrapartum fetal monitoring
- Describe technique of inserting internal monitors during labor
- Describe the complications of internal monitors in labor
- Be able to perform intrapartum fetal monitoring

INTRODUCTION/BACKGROUND

- External monitors are used in labor until indications for internalization of monitoring are present
  - External tocodynamometers measure contraction frequency and duration but cannot measure strength of contractions
  - Fetal scalp electrodes record the fetal heart rate in high-risk pregnancies and in fetuses at risk for hypoxic complications during labor.

UNIVERSAL PRECAUTIONS

- Sterile gloves must be worn while placing internal monitors
- Evaluate the need for face and eye protection as well as a gown.

OBTAIN INFORMED CONSENT

- Introduce yourself to the patient
- Explain the procedure to the patient, as well as the risks and benefits
- Gain informed consent to continue.

INDICATIONS

- When external monitors do not give a clear tracing to determine the relationship between changes in fetal heart rate and contractions

- Intrauterine pressure catheter (IUPC) is a device placed into the amniotic space during labor to measure the uterine contractions strength. It allows an amnioinfusion to be performed in cases with severe variable fetal heart rate decelerations.
- Fetal scalp electrode (FSE) monitors the fetal heart rate directly and continuously during the intrapartum period. Continuous intrapartum monitoring is recommended in high-risk pregnancies, during an IV infusion of Pitocin, and increased risk of prenatal death.

CONTRAINDICATIONS

- Placenta previa
- Vasa previa
- Intact membranes
- Intrauterine pressure catheter
  - Chorioamnionitis
- Fetal scalp electrode
  - Maternal infections like HIV, active HSV, hepatitis B or C, GBS without antibiotics
  - Known fetal coagulation disorder.

COMPLICATIONS

- Infection
- Bleeding
- Injury to nearby structures
  - Placental abruption or laceration
  - Uterine perforation
  - Vaginal or cervical laceration
  - Fetal injury.

BASIC EQUIPMENT

- Sterile gloves
- Sterile water-based lubrication
- Intrauterine pressure cathether
- Fetal scalp electrode
- Appropriate cable connecters.

SITES/POSITIONING

- Patient should be made comfortable
- Most common position is dorsal lithotomy position.

PREPARATION

- Perform a cervical exam prior to placement of either device to confirm that
  - Cervix is dilated
  - Membranes are ruptured
  - The fetus is in vertex position
- Leave dominant hand in place inside the vagina with fingers on the fetal head
- Assistant will be needed to hand you the sterile equipment for internal placement.

IUPC PLACEMENT

- Insert the tip of the introducer inside the cervical os on the side away from the placenta
- If you meet resistance stop and change the angle of the introducer then reattempt insertion
- Hold the introducer in position and thread the catheter through the introducer 10–12 cm. Amniotic fluid should be seen in the catheter
- Once proper position is reached, remove the introducer, attach to cables and secure to the patient's leg. Patient cough should produce a spike in pressure.

FSE PLACEMENT

- Identify the parietal or occipital bone for application of the electrode
- Place the introducer against the fetal head then expose the needle electrode
- Apply pressure to keep the needle against the scalp while rotating the electrode clockwise
- Remove the introducer and attach to mother's leg and monitor cables.

REMOVAL

- To remove the fetal scalp electrode, turn the wires counterclockwise. If the electrode is not coming off, cut the wire and remove after delivery
- Remove the intrauterine pressure catheter by simply pulling the catheter out.

SELF-ASSESSMENT QUIZ

1. Evidence-based data from the literature suggest that:
   a. Continuous fetal monitoring should be used in low-risk women
   b. Continuous fetal monitoring should not be used in low-risk women
   c. All of the above
   d. None of the above
2. Indications for continuous intrapartum fetal monitoring are:
   a. IUGR
   b. Premature rupture of membranes
   c. High-risk pregnancy
   d. Post-term pregnancy
   e. All of the above
   f. None of the above
3. Continuous electronic fetal intrapartum monitoring has been shown to reduce:
   a. Neonatal mortality
   b. Cerebral palsy
   c. All of the above
   d. None of the above
4. Absolute contraindications for use of internal monitors in labor are:
   a. Intact membranes
   b. Placenta previa
   c. Vasa previa
   d. All of the above
   e. None of the above
5. 38-year-old G1P0 is in labor. The physician has prescribed an IV infusion of Pitocin. The physician should ensure that which of the following is implemented before initiating the infusion?
   a. Epidural analgesia
   b. Continuous electronic fetal monitoring
   c. An IV infusion of antibiotic
   d. Placing a code cart at the patient's bedside

Answers

1. b   2. e   3. d   4. d   5. b

SUGGESTED READING

1. Bakker PC, Colenbrander GJ, Verstraeten AA, Van Geijn HP. The quality of intrapartum fetal heart rate monitoring. Eur J Obstet Gynecol Reprod Biol. 2004;116(1):22-7.
2. Cohen WR, Ommani S, Hassan S, Mirza FG, Solomon M, Brown R. Accuracy and reliability of fetal heart rate monitoring using maternal abdominal surface electrodes. Acta Obstet Gynecol Scand. 2012;91(11):1306-13.
3. Dowdle MA. Comparison of two intrauterine pressure catheters during labor. J Reprod Med. 2003;48:501.
4. Euliano TY, Nguyen MT, Darmanjian S, et al. Monitoring uterine activity during labor: A comparison of 3 methods. Am J Obstet Gynecol. 2013;208:66.e1.
5. Harper LM, Shanks AL, Tuuli MG, et al. The risks and benefits of internal monitors in laboring patients. Am J Obstet Gynecol. 2013;209:38.e1.
6. Lind BK. Complications caused by extramembranous placement of intrauterine pressure catheters. Am J Obstet Gynecol. 1999;180:1034.
7. Macones GA, Hankins GD, Spong CY, Hauth J, Moore T. The 2008 National Institute of Child Health and Human Development workshop report on electronic fetal monitoring: Update on definitions, interpretation, and research guidelines. Obstet Gynecol. 2008;112(3):661-6.

Triage OB Ultrasound

Kupesic Plavsic S

OBJECTIVES

- Describe the components of triage OB ultrasound
- Know the indications for limited prenatal ultrasound
- Be able to perform a limited prenatal ultrasound

INTRODUCTION/BACKGROUND

- A limited ultrasound can be performed to evaluate any clinical concern in pregnancy at any gestational age
- When this ultrasound is performed, it does not take the place of the anatomy or dating ultrasounds.

UNIVERSAL PRECAUTIONS

- Gloves must be worn while performing the ultrasound

OBTAIN INFORMED CONSENT

- Introduce yourself to the patient
- Explain the procedure to the patient, as well as the risks and benefits
- Gain informed consent to continue.

INDICATIONS

- Vaginal bleeding
- Pelvic pain
- Suspected rupture of membranes
- Evaluating fetal lie.

CONTRAINDICATIONS

- None.

COMPLICATIONS

• None.

BASIC EQUIPMENT

• Ultrasound machine
• Transducer
• Lubricant
• Towel
• Gloves.

SITES/POSITIONING

• Patients should lie supine
• The ultrasound probe should be positioned parallel to the maternal spine and perpendicular to the floor with each measurement.

PREPARATION

• Gather equipment
• Plug in ultrasound machine and turn it on
• Warm lubricant if desired
• Expose the patient's abdomen
• Protect the patient's pants or undergarments with a towel
• Apply gel to the areas to be examined.

MEASURING AMNIOTIC FLUID INDEX

• Below normal amniotic fluid index may be a sign that the membranes are ruptured
    – Amniotic fluid index (AFI) from 8–18 is normal
• Measure the largest vertical fluid pocket from each of the 4 abdominal quadrants
• Sum the values to get the AFI.

LOCATION OF THE PLACENTA

• Determining the location of the placenta can help to rule out placental reasons as a cause of vaginal bleeding
• Place the ultrasound on the maternal abdomen, looking for the placental location
    – Determine the margin of the placenta
    – Ensure to place the transducer suprapubic to see if the placenta is low-lying, near or in contact with the cervix.

DETERMINING PRESENTING FETAL PART

- Place the transducer low on the maternal abdomen, just suprapubic, to evaluate for the presenting fetal part
- Visualization of the fetal skull confirms that the fetus is vertex.

AFTER THE ULTRASOUND

- Clean the mother's abdomen with the towel
- Allow the mother to cover her abdomen for privacy if desired
- Make sure to clean the transducer probe.

SELF-ASSESSMENT QUIZ

1. List the components of a basic triage OB ultrasound exam:
   a. Assessment of AFI, placental location and presenting fetal part
   b. Assessment of BPD, OFD, HC, AC and FL
   c. Assessment of fetal biometry and Doppler
   d. Assessment of fetal anatomy by 3D ultrasound
2. What are the indications for a basic triage OB ultrasound examination:
   a. Vaginal bleeding   b. Abdominal and pelvic pain
   c. Suspected rupture of membranes   d. All of the above
   e. None of the above
3. Amniotic fluid index is measured:
   a. As the deepest unobstructed maximal vertical length of a single fluid pocket
   b. As a sum of two deepest vertical pockets in upper quadrants of maternal abdomen
   c. As a sum of two deepest vertical pockets in lower quadrants of maternal abdomen
   d. By adding the values of individual amniotic pocket depths in each quadrant
4. Normal amniotic fluid index value ranges:
   a. From 5 to 10 cm   b. From 10 to 20 cm
   c. From 8 to 18 cm   d. From 18 to 28 cm
5. Basic triage ultrasound is performed
   a. Transabdominally   b. Transvaginally
   c. Transperineally   d. Transrectally
   e. Transcervically   f. All of the above

Answers

1. a   2. d   3. d   4. c   5. a

SUGGESTED READING

1. ACOG. Antepartum fetal surveillance. In: Practice Bulletin 9. American College of Obstetrics and Gynecology; October 1999. http://www.acog.org/-/media/List-of-Titles/PB List of Titles. pdf; Accessed on October 2014.

2. ACR-AIUM-ACOG Practice Guidelines for the Performance of Antepartum Obstetrical Ultrasound, Revised 2007. Reston, VA. ACR Standards, Resolution 25.

3. American Institute of Ultrasound in Medicine. AIUM practice guideline for the performance of obstetric ultrasound examinations. J Ultrasound Med. 2010;29(1): 157-66.

4. Brant WE. Obstetric Ultrasound. Fundamentals of Diagnostic Radiology, 3rd Edition. Lippincott Williams and Wilkins: Philadelphia, PA; 2007. p. 976-1001.

5. Guidelines for Professional Working Standards. Ultrasound Practice. United Kingdom Association of Sonographers; October 2008. http://www.sor.org/system/files/document-library/members/sor_D41663_Prof._Guidelines_Booklet.pdf; Accessed on October 2014.

6. Marinac-Dabic D, Krulewitch CJ, Moore RM Jr. The safety of prenatal ultrasound exposure in human studies. Epidemiology. 2002;13:S19-S22.

Normal Vaginal Delivery

Mendez MD, Kupesic Plavsic S

OBJECTIVES

- List the indications and contraindications for normal spontaneous vaginal delivery
- Describe delivery technique
- Describe the complications of vaginal delivery
- Be able to perform normal vaginal delivery

INTRODUCTION/BACKGROUND

- First stage of labor is when cervical changes happen
- Delivery occurs during the second stage of labor, the time between complete cervical dilation to delivery of the infant
- Delivery of the placenta is during the third stage of labor.

UNIVERSAL PRECAUTIONS

- Sterile gloves and sterile gown must be worn while delivering an infant
- Face, eye and shoe protection is highly recommended.

OBTAIN INFORMED CONSENT

- Introduce yourself to the patient
- Explain the delivery procedure to the patient, as well as your role in the delivery
- Informed consent is not needed, but all patients should be educated about their medical care.

INDICATIONS

- Patients in the second stage of labor.

CONTRAINDICATIONS

- Cord prolapse
- Transverse fetal lie
- Breech, face or brow presentation
- Cephalopelvic disproportion
- Macrosomia
- Complete placenta previa
- Vasa previa
- Maternal or fetal instability
- High order births
- Herpes simplex virus with active genital lesions or prodromal symptoms
- Untreated HIV infection.

COMPLICATIONS

- Failure to progress
- Premature rupture of membranes
- Intrapartum or postpartum hemorrhage
- Nonreassuring fetal heart rate
- Retained placenta
- Shoulder dystocia
- Uterine rupture
- Infection
- Bleeding.

BASIC EQUIPMENT

- Skin prep solution, sterile towels and drape
- Water-based lubrication jelly
- Bulb suction, cord clamp, scissors
- 2 hemostats, minilaps
- Specimen container for cord blood
- Tray for placenta.

SITES/POSITIONING

- Patient may choose from multiple positions
    - Lithotomy position: Patient supine with the head of bead elevated and their knees flexed
    - Squatting, kneeling on hands or knees, lying on one side with upper leg supported.

PREPARATION

- Delivery is close when the baby's head causes the perineum to bulge
- At that time, drape under perineum, gown and glove, and may prep skin if desired
- With nondominant hand support the head to keep the head flexed
- With the other hand support the perineum to decrease likelihood of tearing.

PROCEDURE STEPS

- Once the head delivers, check around the neck for the cord with your fingers
    - If present, reduce cords if able. If too tight to reduce, deliver the baby and reduce after delivery
- Place a hand on each side of the baby's face, with the fingers over the cheeks
    - Apply posterior traction on the head until the anterior shoulder delivers
    - Then apply anterior traction to deliver the posterior shoulder
- With one hand still supporting the head, use the other hand to catch the body as it is delivered
- Place the baby on the mother's belly if maternal and fetal status are stable
    - With 2 hemostats (or a hemostat and a cord clamp), clamp the umbilical cord one minute after delivery
    - Allow patient or family to cut cord if desired.

THIRD STAGE

- Collect cord blood in specimen container
- With sterile towel, begin fundal massage
- Watch for signs of placental separation:
    - Lengthening cord, gush of blood, firm fundus
- Apply gentle posterior traction on the cord and gentle suprapubic pressure with the other hand. Control delivery speed
- Inspect placenta for 3 vessel cord and to determine if the placenta is intact.

SELF-ASSESSMENT QUIZ

1. Choose the most accurate option:
   a. The second stage of labor encompasses the onset of labor to the complete dilatation of the cervix
   b. The second stage of labor is divided into latent and active phases
   c. The second stage consists of the time from complete dilatation of the cervix to delivery of the infant
   d. The third stage is complete at the delivery of the placenta

2. Choose the most accurate option:
   a. The practice of routine episiotomy should be abandoned
   b. Antenatal perineal massage increases the risk of episiotomy
   c. Routine episiotomy decreases healing complications and increases the likelihood of maintaining an intact perineum
   d. None of the above

3. Postpartum hemorrhage is defined as:
   a. Excess blood loss from the uterus (more than 1000 mL) during and after delivery
   b. Excess blood loss from the uterus (more than 500 mL) during and after delivery
   c. Between 100 and 300 mL of blood loss during and after delivery
   d. None of the above

4. The most common causes of postpartum hemorrhage are:
   a. Uterine atony   b. Retained products
   c. Trauma to the genital tract   d. Coagulopathies
   e. All of the above   f. None of the above

5. Active management of the third stage of labor includes:
   a. Administration of oxytocin after head delivery, late cord clamping and forced cord traction
   b. Administration of oxytocin after delivery of the anterior shoulder, early cord clamping and controlled cord traction
   c. Administration of oxytocin after delivery of the posterior shoulder, late cord clamping and forced cord traction
   d. None of the above

Answers

1. c   2. a   3. b   4. e   5. b

SUGGESTED READING

1. Andersson O, Hellström-Westas L, Andersson D, Domellöf M. Effect of delayed versus early umbilical cord clamping on neonatal outcomes and iron status at 4 months: A randomised controlled trial. BMJ. 2011;343:d7157.

2. Freeman B, Garite T, Nageotte M. Fetal Heart Rate Monitoring. 3rd. Lippincott Williams & Wilkins; 2003.

3. Gabbe SG, Simpson JL, Niebyl JR, Galan H, Goetzl L, Jauniaux ER, Landon M. Obstetrics: Normal and problem pregnancies. 5th. Philadelphia, Pa: Churchill and Livingstone; 2007.

4. Goetzl LM. ACOG Practice Bulletin. Clinical Management Guidelines for Obstetrician-Gynecologists Number 36, July 2002. Obstetric analgesia and anesthesia. Obstet Gynecol. 2002;100(1):177-91.

5. Kilpatrick S, Garrison E. Normal labor and delivery. In: Gabbe S (Ed). Obstetrics, Normal and Problem Pregnancies. 5th ed. Philadelphia: Churchill Livingston Elsevier; 2007. p. 303-21.

6. National Collaborating Centre for Women's and Children's Health. Intrapartum Care: Care of Healthy Women and Their Babies During Childbirth. London: RCOG Press; 2007.

7. Patterson DA, Winslow M, Matus CD. Spontaneous vaginal delivery. Am Fam Physician. 2008;1:78(3):336-41.

40

CHAPTER

Perineal Laceration Repair

Mendez MD, Kupesic Plavsic S

OBJECTIVES

- Describe perineal laceration repair technique
- Know the indications for perineal laceration repair
- Describe the complications of perineal laceration repair
- Be able to perform perineal laceration repair

INTRODUCTION/BACKGROUND

- The female perineum can be damaged during delivery, sports, and intercourse
  - Superficial lacerations heal spontaneously
- Repairing a deeper perineal laceration provides for hemostasis and reapproximates the tissues.

UNIVERSAL PRECAUTIONS

- Sterile gloves must be worn while suturing
- Evaluate the need for face and eye protection as well as a gown.

OBTAIN INFORMED CONSENT

- Introduce yourself to the patient
- Explain the procedure to the patient, as well as the risks and benefits
- Gain informed consent to continue.

INDICATIONS

- Hemorrhage
- Restore structure and function.

CONTRAINDICATIONS

- Superficial laceration
- Unstable patient.

COMPLICATIONS

- Hematoma
- Infection
- Bleeding.

BASIC EQUIPMENT

- Suture driver, forceps, scissors
- Absorbable suture like 3-0 chromic
- 18 G and 22 G needle
- Lidocaine
- 10 mL syringe
- Skin prep solution.

SITES/POSITIONING

- Place patient supine in the lithotomy position with knees slightly flexed.

PREPARATION

- Clean perineum with skin prep solution
- Draw up lidocaine and infiltrate the laceration to provide local anesthetic.

PROCEDURE STEPS

- Place first stitch 1 cm proximal to apex
- Use continuous stitches to reapproximate tissues and close dead spaces
- Place crown stitch at hymenal ring
- Reapproximate perineal muscles, then close skin with subcuticular stitches and place the final stitch deep to the hymenal ring.

SELF-ASSESSMENT QUIZ

1. Repair of the perineum requires
   a. Good lighting and visualization
   b. Surgical instruments
   c. Suture material
   d. Adequate anesthesia
   e. All of the above
   f. None of the above
2. For effective repair of obstetric perineal laceration a physician should have
   a. Knowledge of perineal anatomy
   b. Appropriate surgical technique
   c. Appropriate surgical instruments
   d. All of the above
   e. None of the above
3. Potential sequelae of obstetric perineal lacerations include
   a. Chronic perineal pain
   b. Urinary incontinence
   c. Fecal incontinence
   d. Chest pain
   e. a + b + c
   f. None of the above
4. The most common complications of perineal lacerations are:
   a. Infection
   b. Dysmenorrhea
   c. Bleeding
   d. Dyspareunia
   e. Hematoma
   f. a + c + e
   g. b + d
5. First stich should be inserted
   a. 1 cm proximal to the apex
   b. 1 cm distal to the apex
   c. 1 cm behind the apex
   d. At the apex
   e. It does not really matter

Answers

1. e   2. d   3. e   4. f   5. a

SUGGESTED READING

1. DeLancey JOL. Surgical Anatomy of the Female Pelvis. In: Rock JA, Jones HW III (Eds). TeLinde's Operative Gynecology, 10th ed; 2008. p. 82-112.
2. Hale RW, Ling FW. Episiotomy: Procedure and Repair Techniques. Washington, DC: American College of Obstetricians and Gynecologists. 2007. p. 1-24.
3. Kilpatrick S, Garrison E. Normal labor and delivery. In: Gabbe S (Ed). Obstetrics, Normal and Problem Pregnancies, 5th ed. Philadelphia: Churchill Livingston Elsevier. 2007. p. 303-21.
4. Ould F. A Treatise on Midwifery in Three Parts. Dublin: Nelson and Connor; 1742.
5. Quilligan EJ, Zuspan F. Douglass-Stromme Operative Obstetrics. 5th ed. Norwalk, CT: Appleton-Century-Crofts; 1988. p. 698.
6. Sleep J, Grant A, Garcia J, Elbourne D, Spencer J, Chalmers D. The West Berkshire perineal management trial. BMJ. 1984;289(6445):587-90.
7. Stein TA, DeLancey JO. Structure of the perineal membrane in females: gross and microscopic anatomy. Obstet Gynecol. 2008;111(3):686-93.

Newborn Circumcision

Prieto Jimenez C

OBJECTIVES

- Describe newborn circumcision technique
- List the indications for circumcision
- Describe the complications of newborn circumcision
- Be able to perform newborn circumcision

INTRODUCTION/BACKGROUND

- Circumcision is the removal of the prepuce—the skin covering the tip of the penis
- Is a fairly common procedure for male newborns.

UNIVERSAL PRECAUTIONS

- Gloves must be worn while performing circumcision
- Evaluate the need for face and eye protection as well as a gown.

OBTAIN INFORMED CONSENT

- Introduce yourself to the parent
- Explain the procedure to the parent, as well as the risks and benefits
- Gain informed consent to continue.

INDICATIONS

- Medical indications
  - Phimosis—prepuce not retractable
  - Paraphimosis—prepuce not reducible
  - Balanitis—infection of glans penis

- Posthitis—infection of prepuce
- Management of recurrent UTIs
- Parental request
  - Religious or cultural preference, tradition, or can be thought to improve hygiene.

CONTRAINDICATIONS

- Penile anomalies
  - Chordee: Curved penis
  - Hypospadias
  - Epispadias
  - Webbed penis
  - Micropenis
  - Buried penis
  - Ambiguous genitalia
- Patient prematurity.

COMPLICATIONS

- Bleeding
- Infection
- Meatal stenosis
- Adhesions
- Wound separation
- Unsatisfactory appearance of scar.

BASIC EQUIPMENT

- 22 gauge needle, 3 cc syringe
- Lidocaine without epinephrine
- Skin prep solution
- Sterile gloves, sterile drape
- 2 hemostats, scissors
- Plastibell device
- Sterile string.

SITES/POSITIONING

- Infant will be positioned prone, naked below the waist
- Arms and legs are restrained, with legs in a spread position to allow visualization of the penis.

PREPARATION

- Ensure the glans and penis are without abnormalities
- Inject lidocaine without epinephrine circumferentially at the base of the penis
- Apply small hemostats to lateral edges of foreskin to allow for a grip
- Estimate the amount of foreskin to be removed.

PROCEDURE STEPS

- Make a cut in the dorsal edge of the prepuce
- Hold the skin open for visualization and bluntly separate the skin layers on the internal edge of the prepuce, separating it from the glans
- Position the Plastibell device between the glans and the prepuce
- Tie sterile string over the foreskin and around the device to cut off the blood supply
- Trim the foreskin tissue
- Remove the end of the bell, leaving the ring.

REMOVAL

- The tissue under the ring will die and slough off, and the ring will come off on its own within 12 days of the circumcision.

SELF-ASSESSMENT QUIZ

1. What allows for the correct placement of the Plastibell device?
   a. Sterile string
   b. Blunt dissection
   c. Cutting a hole in the foreskin
   d. Trimming off the foreskin
2. What is not a medical reason to remove foreskin?
   a. Improved hygiene
   b. Phimosis
   c. Paraphimosis
   d. Balanitis
3. Which is a contraindication for circumcision?
   a. Hypospadias
   b. Epispadias
   c. Patient prematurity
   d. All of the above
4. What would the correct choice be to inject for pain control prior to circumcision?
   a. Solu-Medrol
   b. Lidocaine
   c. Epinephrine
   d. Toradol
5. Which is a not considered a complication of circumcision?
   a. Buried penis
   b. Bleeding
   c. Infection
   d. Meatal stenosis

Answers

1. b   2. a   3. d   4. b   5. a

SUGGESTED READING

1. Alanis MC, Lucidi RS. Neonatal circumcision: A review of the world's oldest and most controversial operation. Obstet Gynecol Surv. 2004;59(5):379-95.
2. Alter GJ, Horton CE, Horton CE Jr. Buried penis as a contraindication for circumcision. J Am Coll Surg. 1994;178(5):487-90.
3. Barrie H, Huntingford PJ, Gough MH. The Plastibell technique for circumcision. Br Med J. 1965;2(5456):273-5.
4. Elder JS. Circumcision. BJU Int. 2007;99(6):1553-64.
5. Lander J, Brady-Fryer B, Metcalfe JB, Nazarali S, Muttitt S. Comparison of ring block, dorsal penile nerve block, and topical anesthesia for neonatal circumcision: A randomized controlled trial. JAMA. 1997;278(24):2157-62.
6. Lannon CM, Bailey AGB, Fleischman AR. Circumcision policy statement. American Academy of Pediatrics. Task Force on Circumcision. Pediatrics. 1999;103(3):686-93.
7. Schoen EJ. Ignoring evidence of circumcision benefits. Pediatrics. 2006;118(1):385-7.

Pap Smear

Kupesic Plavsic S

OBJECTIVES

- Know the indications for Pap testing
- Describe Pap smear technique
- Be able to perform Pap test

INTRODUCTION/BACKGROUND

- The Papanicolaou test collects cells from the cervical transformation zone for microscopic examination to detect lesions
  - New liquid-based cytology places the cell into a vial of liquid for laboratory evaluation
  - Looks for cancerous or precancerous changes.

UNIVERSAL PRECAUTIONS

- Gloves must be worn while performing the Pap test.

OBTAIN INFORMED CONSENT

- Introduce yourself to the patient
- Explain the procedure to the patient, as well as the risks and benefits
- Gain informed consent to continue.

INDICATIONS

- Women over age 21
- Normal screening timeline
  - Women age 21–29 repeat every 3 years
  - Women age 30–65 repeat every 5 years.

CONTRAINDICATIONS

- Women under age 20
- Women with positive results on previous Pap tests may not be on screening timeline.

COMPLICATIONS

- Bleeding
- Infection.

BASIC EQUIPMENT

- Exam table with lithotomy extensions
- Exam gloves
- Large cleaning swab
- Cervical broom or spatula and brush
- Specimen container
- Light source
- Speculum
- Surgilube lubricant.

SITES/POSITIONING

- Patient should lay supine in the dorsal lithotomy position
- The edge of the patient's buttocks should be at the edge of the exam table
- When ready to begin, instruct the patient to relax her legs open and to stay as relaxed as possible.

PREPARATION

- Put on gloves
- Place equipment on a bedside tray and ready equipment for use
  - Open speculum and swabs, ready light source
- Use lukewarm water or minimal surgilube to lubricate the outer edge of the speculum, not at the tip.

PROCEDURE STEPS

- With your nondominant hand spread the labia to visualize the vagina
- Insert the speculum tip with the wide edge oriented anteroposteriorly
- Advance the speculum and open the blades when the speculum is fully inserted
- Ensure that the cervix is visualized between the blades
- Clean discharge from the cervix with swab.

SPECIMEN COLLECTION

- Based on the collection equipment
  - Cervical broom: Place the long tip of the broom in the cervical os and rotate 5 times on the surface of the cervix
  - Cervical spatula and brush: Rotate the spatula 360 degrees, then insert the brush into the cervical os and rotate the brush 180 degrees
- Place specimens in container and break off the removable heads of the devices.

SELF-ASSESSMENT QUIZ

1. You are performing an annual pelvic exam of a 22-year-old patient. How often does she need a Pap test?
    - a. Every year
    - b. Every two years
    - c. Every three years
    - d. Every five years
2. When can a patient stop getting Pap?
    - a. At age of 55
    - b. At age of 60
    - c. At age of 65
    - d. At age of 70
3. The physician asks a resident to position a patient for a Pap smear. Which of the following positions is normally used for this procedure?
    - a. Dorsal recumbent position
    - b. Lithotomy position
    - c. Left lateral position
    - d. Right lateral position
4. Pap test is used mainly to detect
    - a. Ovarian cancer
    - b. Patency of the Fallopian tube
    - c. Uterine fibroid
    - d. Cervical cancer
5. Which of the following is correct concerning the performance of a Pap test?
    - a. The patient should not douche or use vaginal creams for at least 2 days before the test
    - b. The patient should not have intercourse for at least 7 days before the test
    - c. The patient should not use IUD
    - d. None of the above

Answers

1. c   2. c   3. b   4. d   5. a

SUGGESTED READING

1. Kulasingam SL, Havrilesky L, Ghebre R, Myers ER. Screening for cervical cancer: A decision analysis for the U.S. Preventive Services Task Force. AHRQ Publication No. 11-05157-EF-1. Rockville, MD: Agency for Healthcare Research and Quality; 2011.
2. Marchand L, Mundt M, Klein G, Agarwal SC. Optimal collection technique and devices for a quality pap smear. WMJ. 2005;104:51-5.
3. NIH Consensus Statement: Cervical Cancer. National Institutes of Health. 1996. p. 1-38.
4. Sasieni P, Castanon A. Call and recall cervical screening programme: Screening interval and age limits. Curr Diagn Pathol. 2006;12:114-26.
5. Saslow D, Solomon D, Lawson HW, Killackey M, Kulasingam SL, Cain J, et al. American Cancer Society, American Society for Colposcopy and Cervical Pathology, and American Society for Clinical Pathology screening guidelines for the prevention and early detection of cervical cancer. CA Cancer J Clin. 2012;62(3):147-71. DOI: 10.3322/caac.21139. Epub 2012 Mar 14.
6. Screening for Cervical Cancer: Clinical Summary of U.S. Preventive Services Task Force Recommendation. AHRQ Publication No. 11-05156-EF-3, March 2012. http://www.uspreventiveservicestaskforce.org/uspstf11/cervcancer/cervcancersum.htm; Accessed July 2014.

Wet Mount and Whiff Test

Kupesic Plavsic S

INTRODUCTION/BACKGROUND

- All women presenting with abnormal vaginal discharge should have a thorough pelvic examination
- The wet mount test can reveal motility, clue cells or yeast forms
- The Whiff test reveals an amine, fishy odor in patients with trichomoniasis and bacterial vaginosis.

UNIVERSAL PRECAUTIONS

- Gloves must be worn while performing the test and while in contact with the microscope slide
- Evaluate the need for face and eye protection.

OBTAIN INFORMED CONSENT

- Introduce yourself to the patient
- Explain the procedure to the patient, as well as the risks and benefits
- Gain informed consent to continue.

INDICATIONS

- Abnormal vaginal discharge
- Abnormal genital odor
- Genital burning
- Genital itching

CONTRAINDICATIONS

- None.

COMPLICATIONS

- None.

BASIC EQUIPMENT

- Gloves
- Lubricating gel
- Sterile speculum
- Sterile swab
- Sterile saline in a specimen tube
- KOH in a specimen tube
- Microscope slide and coverslip.

SITES/POSITIONING

- Patient should be in the dorsal lithotomy position.

PREPARATION

- Lubricate the outer edges of the speculum, and insert the speculum
- Ensure that the cervix is visualized between the blades
  - If the vaginal discharge is colored, malodorous or is an increased amount, then vaginitis is likely
  - If the cervix is friable, edematous, or erythematous, then cervicitis is likely.

PROCEDURE STEPS

- Take two swab samples of the vaginal vault and vaginal wall
- Place the swabs in the test tube with 0.5 mL of sterile saline
- Remove the speculum
- Perform a bimanual examination looking for cervical tenderness or enlargement of the uterus or adnexa.

SAMPLE ANALYSIS

- **Wet mount**: Place a drop of vaginal discharge on a slide with 1–2 drops of 0.9% isotonic NaCl solution, cover with a cover slip and examine microscopically under high power (400x). Identify clue cells, WBC, RBC, bacteria, yeast, hyphae, or motility
- **Whiff test**: Place a drop of vaginal discharge on a slide with 10% KOH solution. A positive test result is the release of an amine, fishy odor after the addition of KOH to the discharge.

SELF-ASSESSMENT QUIZ

1. What are the most common causes of vaginitis?
   a. Bacterial vaginosis
   b. Trichomoniasis
   c. Vulvovaginal candidiasis
   d. All of the above
   e. None of the above
2. Typical signs of bacterial vaginosis are:
   a. Positive Whiff test
   b. Milky discharge
   c. Presence of clue cells on microscopic examination of vaginal fluid
   d. Trichomonads visualized microscopically in saline
   e. All of the above
   f. a + b + c
   g. a + b + d
3. Typical signs of trichomoniasis are:
   a. Positive Whiff test
   b. Leukocytes more numerous than epithelial cells
   c. Presence of clue cells on microscopic examination of vaginal fluid
   d. Trichomonads visualized microscopically in saline
   e. All of the above
   f. a + b + c
   g. a + b +d
4. Typical signs of vaginal candidiasis are:
   a. Positive Whiff test
   b. Leukocytes more numerous than epithelial cells
   c. Budding yeast on microscopic examination of vaginal fluid with a 10% KOH
   d. Trichomonads visualized microscopically in saline
   e. All of the above
   f. a + b + c
   g. a + b + d
5. Symptoms of vaginitis may be associated with:
   a. Infection
   b. Atrophic changes
   c. All of the above
   d. None of the above

Answers

1. d   2. f   3. g   4. c   5. c

SUGGESTED READING

1. Croft AC, Woods GL. Specimen collection and handling for diagnosis of infectious diseases. In: McPherson RA, Pincus MR, eds. Henry's Clinical Diagnosis and Management by Laboratory Methods. 22nd ed. Philadelphia, Pa: Elsevier–Saunders; 2011. Chap 63.

2. Eckert LO, Lentz GM. Infections of the lower and upper genital tracts: Vulva, vagina, cervix, toxic shock syndrome, endometritis, and salpingitis. In: Lentz GM, Lobo RA, Gershenson DM, Katz VL. (Eds). Comprehensive Gynecology. 6th ed. Philadelphia, Pa: Elsevier Mosby; 2012. Chap 23.

3. Hobbs M, Sena EC, Swygard H, Schwebke J. Trichomonas vaginalis and Trichomoniasis. In: KK Holmes, PF Sparling, WE Stamm, P Piot, JN Wasserheit, L Corey, MS Cohen, DH Watts (eds). Sexually Transmitted Diseases, 4th edition. New York: McGraw-Hill; 2008. p. 771-93.

4. Katz VL, Lentz GM, Lobo RA, Gershenson DM. Comprehensive Gynecology. 5th ed. Mosby; 2007. p. 598-600.

5. Low N, Cowan F. Genital chlamydial infection. Clin Evid; 2003;(9):1721-8.

6. Mass D. Ensuring Correct Diagnosis in Testing for Vaginitis. Medical Office Report. 1998;11(3):2-3.

7. Owen KO, Clenney TL. Management of vaginitis. Am Family Physician. 2004;1:70(11):2125-32.

8. Soper DE. Sexually transmitted disease and pelvic inflammatory disease. Primary Care of Women. 1995. p. 339-47.

44

CHAPTER

Pessary Fitting

Kupesic Plavsic S

OBJECTIVES

- Know the indications for the use of pessary
- Describe sizing technique for pessary placement
- Describe the complications of pessary use
- Be able to perform pessary sizing and placement

INTRODUCTION/BACKGROUND

- Pessaries can be used to provide structural support to the pelvic organs
- Pessaries should be chosen and sized to improve prolapse symptoms, decrease complications and decrease discomfort
- Symptoms include pelvic pressure, vaginal bulge, difficulties with urination or defecation or dyspareunia.

UNIVERSAL PRECAUTIONS

- Gloves must be worn while sizing and fitting the pessary
- Evaluate the need for face and eye protection as well as a gown.

OBTAIN INFORMED CONSENT

- Introduce yourself to the patient
- Explain the procedure to the patient, as well as the risks and benefits
- Gain informed consent to continue.

INDICATIONS

- Urinary bladder prolapse
- Uterine prolapse
- Rectocele
- Urinary incontinence
- Poor surgical candidate

CONTRAINDICATIONS

- Vaginal ulceration
- Severe vaginal atrophy
- Vaginal infection.

COMPLICATIONS

- New difficulties in emptying bowel or bladder
- Discomfort
- Pressure
- Pain
- Vaginal ulceration
- Infection.

BASIC EQUIPMENT

- Basic support requiring introitus strength
  - Ring or donut
- Self-retaining if introitus musculature not tight
  - Gellhorn or cube
- Urinary incontinence
  - Incontinence ring
- Gloves
- Lubrication.

SITES/POSITIONING

- Patient should be in the dorsal lithotomy position for sizing and fitting.

PREPARATION

- Assess for pelvic muscle tone, support and patency of introitus with a digital pelvic examination
- Digital measurements:
  - Vaginal length from posterior symphysis to posterior fornix (length of gellhorn neck)
  - Vaginal width at the apex (diameter of pessary)
  - Diameter of the introitus and vaginal shaft (cube size).

PROCEDURE STEPS

- Choose the pessary style based on indication and introitus patency
- Choose size based on measurements from digital pelvic exam
- Lubricate the vagina, apply pressure to bend the pessary and insert through the introitus while applying perineal pressure
- This pessary lies behind the symphysis and can lie as high as the posterior fornix.

VERIFY PESSARY FIT

- To check fit, have the patient in Valsalva maneuver
  - May advance toward the introitus with pressure, but it should not be expelled
  - If expelled use a larger size or another style
- Have the patient perform normal activity like walking, bending, standing or sitting
  - If the pessary is uncomfortable or the patient feels pressure, try a smaller size or different style. Successfully sized, the pessary should be comfortable.

REMOVAL

- Lubricate the introitus
- Place a gloved digit through the finger-size hole or at a hinge notch
- Rotate the pessary to bring the hinge anteriorly to the introitus, and gently pull downward, diagonally, and out
- The vaginal walls will help to fold the pessary as it exits.

SELF-ASSESSMENT QUIZ

1. What is the most efficient size of the pessary?
   a. The smallest one that the patient can wear comfortably
   b. The largest one that the patient can wear comfortably
   c. Size is not important
   d. None of the above
2. Pessaries are fit by trial and error. The physician should, therefore, start with:
   a. The smallest size available   b. The biggest size available
   c. An average sized pessary   d. None of the above
3. Following insertion in a patient with stress incontinence, the physician should check the functionality of the pessary by:
   a. Asking patient to dance to test for any leakage of urine
   b. Asking patient to cough to test for any leakage of urine
   c. Asking patient to stand up to test for any leakage of urine
   d. None of the above
4. Contraindications for the use of pessary are:
   a. Active infections of the vagina
   b. Pelvic inflammatory disease
   c. Noncompliant patient unlikely to follow-up
   d. An allergy to silicone and latex
   e. All of the above
5. Five days after initial fitting of the pessary, a 67-year-old patient, G5 P414 presents with symptoms of vaginal irritation. What is the most appropriate next step?
   a. Perform vaginal examination in speculum and assess the vagina for pressure sores and/or allergic reaction
   b. Explain the patient that this is an expected reaction and that she should not worry
   c. Ask the patient to follow-up in three months
   d. Perform Pap smear

Answers

1. b   2. c   3. b   4. e   5. a

SUGGESTED READING

1. American College of Obstetricians and Gynecologists (ACOG). Pelvic organ prolapse ACOG Practice Bulletin No. 85. 2007;110:717-29.
2. Fernando RJ, Thakar R, Sultan AH, Shah SM, Jones PW. Effect of vaginal pessaries on symptoms associated with pelvic organ prolapse. Obstet Gynecol. 2006;108(1):93-9.
3. Komesu YM, Rogers RG, Rode MA, Craig EC, Gallegos KA, Montoya AR, et al. Pelvic floor symptom changes in pessary users. Am J Obstet Gynecol. 2007;197,620.e1-620.e6.
4. Maito JM, Quam ZA, Craig E, Danner KA, Rogers RG. Predictors of successful pessary fitting and continued use in a nurse-midwifery pessary clinic. Midwif Women's Health. 2006;51(2):78-84.
5. Nyguyen JN, Jones CR. Pessary treatment of pelvic relaxation: Factors affecting successful fitting and continued use. Journal of Wound Ostomy and Continence Nursing. 2005;32(4):255-61.
6. Weber AM, Richter HE. Pelvic organ prolapse. Obstet Gynecol. 2005;106(3):615-34.
7. Wu V, Farrell SA, Baskett TF, Flowerdew G. A simplified protocol for pessary management. Obstet Gynecol. 1997;90(6):990-4.

Bartholin's Cyst Management

Kupesic Plavsic S

OBJECTIVES

- Describe management options for symptomatic Bartholin's cyst
- List the indications for Word catheter placement
- Describe the complications of Bartholin's cyst management
- Be able to perform Word catheter placement

INTRODUCTION/BACKGROUND

- Bartholin glands provide vestibular moisture and may become cystic or abscessed
- Incision and drainage (I and D) is not the preferred procedure as there is a high incidence of recurrence following I and D
  - Obstruction of the duct can lead to cyst formation. Asymptomatic cysts do not need to be treated
  - If the gland becomes infected this may lead to an abscess.

UNIVERSAL PRECAUTIONS

- Gloves must be worn while performing this procedure
- Evaluate the need for face and eye protection as well as a gown.

OBTAIN INFORMED CONSENT

- Introduce yourself to the patient
- Explain the procedure to the patient, as well as the risks and benefits
- Gain informed consent to continue.

INDICATIONS

- Symptomatic Bartholin's cyst
- Bartholin's abscess

CONTRAINDICATIONS

- None.

COMPLICATIONS

- Infection
- Bleeding
- Scar formation
- Cyst recurrence.

BASIC EQUIPMENT

- Nonsterile gloves
- Povidone-iodine swabs
- Sterile gloves and sterile drape
- 1% Lidocaine, 5 mL syringe, 30 g needle
- Word catheter
- 3 mL saline, 3 mL syringe, 25 gauge needle
- Forceps, hemostats
- No 11 scalpel
- 4 × 4 sterile gauze.

SITES/POSITIONING

- The patient should be laying supine in the dorsal lithotomy position.

PREPARATION

- Inflate the catheter to test balloon patency. Deflate catheter to prepare for procedure
- Don nonsterile gloves and clean area with the iodine swabs
- Administer up to 3 mL of lidocaine for local anesthetic to numb the site
- Put on sterile gloves and drape the area.

PROCEDURE STEPS

- Grasp the wall of the cyst or abscess with the forceps in the introitus
- With the other hand use the scalpel to make a 0.5 cm stab incision in the wall
- Drain the contents, if needed break up loculations with the hemostats
- Place the word catheter tip in the incision and inflate catheter with saline
  - Tuck other end of the catheter into the vagina.

SPECIMEN ANALYSIS

- If desired, the contents removed can be sent to the lab for culture or analysis.

POST-PROCEDURE

- The patient should wear an absorbent pad in case of discharge; pelvic rest and sitz baths are recommended for first 2 days
- Broad-spectrum antibiotics may be started if there is a risk of complicated infection.

REMOVAL

- The catheter is left in place for 4–6 weeks in order to create an epithelialized drainage tract
- When the tract appears epithelialized, remove the catheter by deflating the balloon tip.

SELF-ASSESSMENT QUIZ

1. Bartholin's cysts and abscesses are common problems in
   - a. Adolescent patients
   - b. Reproductive age women
   - c. Perimenopausal women
   - d. Postmenopausal women
2. Bartholin's cysts are usually
   - a. Less than 0.5 cm in size
   - b. Less than 1 cm in size
   - c. Between 1 and 3 cm in size
   - d. Larger than 4 cm in size
3. The most common symptoms of Bartholin's cyst enlargement and abscess are
   - a. Vulvar pain
   - b. Dyspareunia
   - c. Inability to engage in sport
   - d. Pain during walking
   - e. All of the above
4. Following the placement of the word catheter, the patient is asked to
   - a. Walk as much as possible to assure correct placement of the catheter
   - b. Undergo pelvic rest until removal of the catheter
   - c. Abstain from sexual intercourse
   - d. a + c
   - e. b + c
5. The word catheter is usually left in place for
   - a. 1 week
   - b. 2 weeks
   - c. 4–6 weeks
   - d. 8 weeks

Answers

1. b   2. c   3. e   4. e   5. c

SUGGESTED READING

1. Aghajanian A, Bernstein L, Grimes DA. Bartholin's duct abscess and cyst: A case-control study. South Med J. 1994;87:26-9.

2. Apgar BS. Bartholin's cyst/abscess: Word catheter insertion. In: Pfenninger JL, Fowler GC (Eds). Procedures for primary care physicians. St. Louis: Mosby; 1994. p. 596-600.

3. Hill DA, Lense JJ. Office management of Bartholin gland cysts and abscesses. Am Fam Physician. 1998;57:1611.

4. Kaufman RH. Benign diseases of the vulva and vagina. 4th ed. St Louis: Mosby; 1994. p. 168-248.

5. Omole F, Simmons BJ, Hacker Y. Management of Bartholin's duct cyst and gland abscess. Am Fam Physician. 2003;68:135.

6. Stenchever MA. Comprehensive Gynecology. 4th ed. St. Louis: Mosby; 2001:482-6, 645-6.

7. Stillman FH, Muto MG. The vulva. In: Ryan KJ, Berkowitz RS, Barbieri RL (Eds). Kistner's Gynecology: Principles and practice. 6th ed. St. Louis: Mosby; 1995. p. 66-8.

8. Wilkinson EJ, Stone IK. Atlas of vulvar disease. 5th ed. Baltimore: Williams and Wilkins; 1995. p. 11-5.

Cervical Polyp Removal

Kupesic Plavsic S

INTRODUCTION/BACKGROUND

- Cervical polyps are common benign cervical growths
  - Caused by focal hyperplasia
  - Usually asymptomatic, however can cause abnormal vaginal bleeding, infections, postcoital spotting and/or leukorrhea
- Polyps may be visualized by speculum exam or felt with bimanual pelvic exam.

UNIVERSAL PRECAUTIONS

- Gloves must be worn while performing the procedure
- Evaluate the need for face and eye protection.

OBTAIN INFORMED CONSENT

- Introduce yourself to the patient
- Explain the procedure to the patient, as well as the risks and benefits
- The patient should be educated that she may bleed after the procedure and should be instructed to wear a pad after the procedure
- Gain informed consent to continue.

INDICATIONS

- Abnormal vaginal bleeding

- Vaginal discharge
- Infertility.

CONTRAINDICATIONS

- Asymptomatic polyps
- Large polyps with a thick base may require surgical removal
  - Surgical dilation and curettage
  - Excision by electrocautery
  - Hysteroscopic removal.

COMPLICATIONS

- Bleeding
- Infection
- Vasovagal response.

BASIC EQUIPMENT

- Ring forceps
- Lubrication
- Sterile speculum
- Large vaginal swab
- Light source
- Silver nitrate stick.

SITES/POSITIONING

- Patient should be placed in the dorsal lithotomy position for ease of visualization.

PREPARATION

- Upon initial exam of the polyp, determine the size and the width of the stalk
  - Do not attempt the removal if the polyp is too large to grasp with ring forceps or if there is a wide base
- Put on gloves
- Place equipment on a bedside tray and ready equipment for use
  - Open speculum and swabs, ready light source.

PROCEDURE STEPS

- Lubricate the speculum and with your nondominant hand spread the labia to visualize the vagina
- Insert the speculum tip with the wide edge oriented anteroposteriorly
- Advance the speculum and open the blades when the speculum is fully inserted

- Ensure that the cervix is visualized between the blades
- Clean discharge from the cervix and the polyp base with swab
- Grasp the polyp with the ring forceps as close to the base as possible
- Twist the polyp until it comes off
- If there is bleeding at the site stop the bleeding by applying the silver nitrate.

SELF-ASSESSMENT QUIZ

1. The most common symptoms of cervical polyps are:
   a. Abnormal vaginal bleeding
   b. Postcoital spotting
   c. Leukorrhea (white or yellow mucous discharge
   d. All of the above
   e. None of the above
2. Cervical polyps are visualized as
   a. Ulcerous cervical lesions   b. Heterogeneous myometrial lesions
   c. Fingerlike growth on the cervix d. Cystic cervical lesions
3. Majority of the polyps are:
   a. Benign (noncancerous)
   b. Cancerous
   c. At high-risk of malignant changes and should be removed
   d. Ulcerous lesions
4. Polyps are typically removed by
   a. Electrocauterization   b. Hysterectomy
   c. Hysterotomy   d. Gentle twisting
5. The most common complication of cervical polyp removal is:
   a. Cancerous changes   b. Bleeding
   c. Ulceration   d. None of the above

Answers

1. d   2. c   3. a   4. d   5. b

SUGGESTED READING

1. Aaro LA, Jacobson LJ, Soule EH. Endocervical polyps. Obstet Gynecol. 1963;21: 659-65.
2. Berzolla CE, Schnatz PF, O'Sullivan DM, et al. Dysplasia and malignancy in endocervical polyps. J Womens Health. 2007;16(9):1317-21.
3. Katz VL. Benign gynecologic lesions. In: Lobo RA, Gershenson DM, Katz VL, (Eds). Comprehensive Gynecology. 6th ed. Philadelphia, Pa: Mosby Elsevier; 2012.
4. Stamatellos I, Stamatopoulos P, Bontis J. The role of hysteroscopy in the current management of the cervical polyps. Arch Gynecol Obstet. 2007;276(4):299-303.

Cervical Colposcopy

Kupesic Plavsic S

INTRODUCTION/BACKGROUND

- Colposcopy provides direct visualization of the cervix
  - Closely examines the cervix under lighted microscopy.

UNIVERSAL PRECAUTIONS

- Gloves must be worn while performing colposcopy
- Evaluate the need for face and eye protection.

OBTAIN INFORMED CONSENT

- Introduce yourself to the patient
- Explain the procedure to the patient, as well as the risks and benefits
- Gain informed consent to continue.

INDICATIONS

- Abnormal Pap smear cytology
- Evaluate cervical lesions
- Cervical polyps
- Cervical warts
- Evaluate patients with history of intrauterine DES exposure as a fetus.

CONTRAINDICATIONS

- None.

COMPLICATIONS

- Bleeding
- Pain
- Infection
- Inability to locate the lesion.

BASIC EQUIPMENT

- Exam table with lithotomy extensions
- Sterile and nonsterile gloves
- Large cleaning swab, sterile saline
- 3–5% acetic acid, Lugol's solution
- Speculum, lubricant gel, specimen jar
- Cervical punch biopsy forceps
- Cytobrush
- Silver nitrate.

SITES/POSITIONING

- Patient is positioned supine in the dorsal lithotomy position.

PREPARATION

- Examine the external genitalia for lesions
- Insert the lubricated speculum through the introitus and position the speculum to visualize the cervix
- If needed, clean the cervix with large cotton swab moistened with saline.

PROCEDURE STEPS

- Apply acetic acid on a large cotton swab and keep in place for at least 60 seconds
  - Reapply if needed in 3–5 minutes
- Position the colposcope to focus on the cervix and the entire transformation zone
  - Document any acetowhite lesions or areas of abnormal vascular patterns
- If no lesions are visible apply Lugol solution to the cervix (dilute iodine)

- Areas with the highest degree of abnormality should be biopsied
  - Topical anesthetic is not required but may be used especially with multiple biopsies
- Following the biopsies, an endocervical sampling is often performed
  - Endocervical curettage should not be performed in pregnancy
- Stop bleeding with silver nitrate if needed
- Remove the speculum.

SELF-ASSESSMENT QUIZ

1. The most common indication for colposcopy is:
   a. Abnormal Pap test result to determine the biopsy site(s) for histologic evaluation
   b. Evaluation of cervical warts
   c. Evaluation of cervical polyps
   d. None of the above
2. The standard methods of colposcopy evaluation include:
   a. Assessment of septa, papillae and solid parts of a cervical lesion
   b. Assessment of color, vessels and margins of a cervical lesion
   c. Assessment of giant cells with shriveled membranes and enlarged nuclei
   d. None of the above
3. At the time of colposcopy the physician should perform:
   a. Single colposcopy directed cervical biopsy
   b. Multiple colposcopy directed cervical biopsies
   c. Random cervical biopsies
   d. None of the above
4. Accuracy of colposcopy is increased when biopsy is performed by
   a. Traditional inspection of cervical lesions
   b. Random identification of cervical lesions
   c. Identifying acetowhite lesions
   d. All of the above
   e. None of the above
5. Colposcopy can also be used for
   a. Diagnosing free fluid in the cul-de-sac
   b. Screening for ovarian cancer
   c. Screening for endometrial cancer
   d. Documenting sexual abuse
   e. None of the above

Answers

1. a   2. b   3. b   4. c   5. d

SUGGESTED READING

1. ACOG Practice Bulletin. Clinical Management Guidelines for Obstetrician-Gynecologists. Human papillomavirus. Obstet Gynecol. 2005;105(4):905-18.
2. Chase D, Kalouyan M, DiSaia P. Colposcopy to evaluate abnormal cervical cytology in 2008. Am J Obstet Gynecol. 2009;200(5):472-80.
3. Kyrgiou M, Tsoumpou I, Vrekoussis T, Martin-Hirsch P, Arbyn M, Prendiville W, et al. The up-to-date evidence on colposcopy practice and treatment of cervical intraepithelial neoplasia: the Cochrane colposcopy and cervical cytopathology collaborative group (C5 group) approach. Cancer Treat Rev. 2006;32:516-23.
4. Noller K, Wagner A Jr. Colposcopy. In: Sciarra JL, ed. Gynecology and Obstetrics. Vol 1. Philadelphia, Pa: Lippincott, Williams and Wilkins; 2000.
5. Saslow D, Solomon D, Lawson HW, Killackey M, Kulasingam SL, Cain J, et al. American Cancer Society, American Society for Colposcopy and Cervical Pathology, and American Society for Clinical Pathology screening guidelines for the prevention and early detection of cervical cancer. CA Cancer J Clin. 2012;62:147-72.
6. Wright TC Jr, Massad LS, Dunton CJ, Spitzer M, Wilkinson EJ, Solomon D; 2006 ASCCP-Sponsored Consensus Conference. 2006 consensus guidelines for the management of women with abnormal cervical screening tests. J Low Genit Tract Dis. 2007;11:201-22.

Endometrial Biopsy

Kupesic Plavsic S

OBJECTIVES

- Be able to describe endometrial biopsy technique
- Be aware of the indications for endometrial biopsy
- Describe the complications of endometrial biopsy
- Know how to perform endometrial biopsy

INTRODUCTION/BACKGROUND

- An endometrial biopsy obtains a tissue sample from the lining of the uterus for histologic examination.

UNIVERSAL PRECAUTIONS

- Gloves must be worn while performing this procedure
- Evaluate the need for face and eye protection.

OBTAIN INFORMED CONSENT

- Introduce yourself to the patient
- Explain the procedure to the patient, as well as the risks and benefits
- Make sure the patient knows that she may bleed or have abdominal cramping after the procedure
- Gain informed consent to continue.

INDICATIONS

- Abnormal menstrual bleeding
- Postmenopausal bleeding
- Amenorrhea
- Excluding presence of endometrial cancer or its precursors
- Perform endometrial dating.

- Evaluate uterine response to hormone therapy
- Assess patients with fertility problems.

CONTRAINDICATIONS

- Pregnancy
- Acute pelvic inflammatory disease
- Acute cervical or vaginal infections
- Clotting disorders
- Cervical obstruction.

COMPLICATIONS

- Bleeding
- Pelvic infection
- Uterine perforation
- Uterine cramping.

BASIC EQUIPMENT

- Nonsterile tray
  - Nonsterile gloves
  - Lubricating gel
  - Absorbent pad
  - Formalin container
- Have available but do not open until needed
  - Sterile cervical dilators
- Sterile tray
  - Sterile vaginal speculum
  - Sterile 4 × 4 gauze
  - Endometrial suction catheter
  - Uterine sound
  - Ring forceps
  - Cervical tenaculum
  - Sterile metal basin with sterile cotton balls soaked in povidone-iodine.

SITES/POSITIONING

- Patient should be supine in dorsal lithotomy position.

PREPARATION

- Have the patient empty her bladder completely
- Perform a bimanual exam with nonsterile gloves to check angulation, size and shape

- Insert speculum and clean cervix using forceps and cotton soaked with iodine.

PROCEDURE STEPS

- Apply sterile gloves
- Apply the tenaculum to the anterior lip of the cervix and hold light retraction
- Insert the uterine sound through the cervical os
  - Average lengths are 6–8 cm
  - If sound is not advancing, consider cervical dilators
- Insert the endometrial biopsy catheter through the cervical os. Withdraw the inner piston
  - While keeping the catheter tip inside the os, twist and move the catheter up and down with at least 4 passes for tissue collection
- Withdraw the catheter and expel the tissue into the specimen container
- A second pass may be performed
- Remove the tenaculum
- Hold pressure on the cervix with gauze if the tenaculum sites are bleeding

SELF-ASSESSMENT QUIZ

1. Endometrial biopsy is useful in work-up of:
   a. Abnormal uterine bleeding   b. Infertility
   c. Cancer screening   d. Endometrial dating
   e. All of the above   f. None of the above
2. Contraindications for endometrial biopsy are:
   a. Pregnancy   b. Pelvic inflammatory disease
   c. Cervical stenosis   d. Endometrial polyp
   e. a + b + c   f. a + b + d
3. If uterine sound will not pass the internal cervical os, the physician should consider:
   a. Placement of hysteroscope
   b. Placement of speculum
   c. Placement of small cervical dilators
   d. Performing saline infusion sonography
4. While performing endometrial biopsy the internal piston of the catheter is fully withdrawn when the catheter is:
   a. Within the cervix   b. Within the vagina
   c. Within the uterine cavity   d. Within the peritoneal cavity
5. The catheter tip is moved in and out using a 360-degrees twisting motion within the uterine cavity:
   a. For at least two excursions between the fundus and the internal cervical os
   b. For at least four excursions between the fundus and the internal cervical os
   c. For at least two excursions between the anterior and posterior uterine wall
   d. For at least four excursions between the anterior and posterior uterine wall

Answers

1. e   2. e   3. c   4. c   5. b

SUGGESTED READING

1. Baughan DM. Office endometrial aspiration biopsy. Fam Pract Res. 1993;15:45-55.
2. Bremer CC. Endometrial biopsy. Female Patient. 1992;17:15-28.
3. Kaunitz AM. Endometrial sampling in menopausal patients. Menopausal Med. 1993;1:5-8.
4. Mettlin C, Jones G, Averette H, Gusberg SB, Murphy GP. Defining and updating the American Cancer Society Guidelines for the cancer-related check-up: Prostate and endometrial cancers. CA Cancer J Clin. 1993;43:42-6.
5. Nesse RE. Managing abnormal vaginal bleeding. Postgrad Med. 1991;89:208;213-4.
6. Reagan MA, Isaacs JH. Office diagnosis of endometrial carcinoma. Prim Care Cancer. 1992;12:49-52.
7. Rutherford T, Auerbach, R. Endometrial Biopsy: A Review of Sampling Techniques. Cooper Surgical Product Bulletin; 2012.
8. Zuber TJ. Endometrial biopsy. Am Fam Physician. 2001;15(63):1131-5.

Dilation and Curettage

Kupesic Plavsic S

OBJECTIVES

- Describe how dilation and curettage (D and C) is performed
- List the indications for D and C procedure
- Describe the complications of D and C
- Be able to perform D and C procedure

INTRODUCTION/BACKGROUND

- Dilation is the opening of the cervix, while curettage is the removal of tissue from the uterine cavity.

UNIVERSAL PRECAUTIONS

- Gloves must be worn while performing dilation and curettage
- Evaluate the need for face and eye protection as well as a gown.

OBTAIN INFORMED CONSENT

- Introduce yourself to the patient
- Explain the procedure to the patient, as well as the risks and benefits
- Gain informed consent to continue.

INDICATIONS

- Abnormal uterine bleeding
- Retained products of conception
- Evaluation of intracavitary findings from imaging procedures
- Insufficient material obtained by office endometrial biopsy
- Endometrial sampling
- Elective abortion
- Treatment and evaluation of gestational trophoblastic disease.

CONTRAINDICATIONS

- Acute pelvic infections
- Pregnancy unless termination desired
- Coagulopathy
- Obstructed vagina and/or cervix
- Inability to visualize cervical os.

COMPLICATIONS

- Bleeding
- Infection
- Cervical laceration
- Uterine perforation
- Intrauterine adhesions
- Bowel injury
- Bladder injury.

BASIC EQUIPMENT

- Cleansing solution, sterile drape
- Foley catheter kit, silver nitrate sticks
- Sterile speculum, lubrication gel
- Tenaculum
- Ring forceps
- 4 × 4 gauze
- 10 mL syringe, 22 g spinal needle, lidocaine
- Cervical dilators
- Uterine sound
- Sharp endometrial curette
- Endometrial suction curette
- Tubing and suction machine

SITES/POSITIONING

- Patient should be supine in dorsal lithotomy position
- She should be at the edge of the examination table with her legs up in stirrups for ease of evaluation.

PREPARATION

- Perform bimanual examination to evaluate uterine size, shape and fundal location
- Clean and drape external genitalia and perineum and insert Foley catheter
- Insert speculum and clean cervix using forceps and cotton soaked with iodine

- Don sterile gloves and place tenaculum on the anterior lip of the cervix
    - Hold light retraction.

PROCEDURE STEPS

- Perform paracervical block
    - 4-site: inject 5 mL at 3, 6, 9 and 12 o'clock where cervix transitions to vaginal wall
- Obtain information about the uterine size using a uterine sound
- If the cervical os is not dilated use dilators
- Choose suction curette based on uterine size from bimanual exam
    - i.e. 10 week size uterus is a size 10 curette
- Insert the cervical curette into the cervix with suction valve off
- Turn on suction and rotate curette 360 degrees inside the uterus continuously until there is no more aspirate
    - Remove suction curette without touching vaginal walls
- May perform sharp endometrial curettage
- Remove tenaculum, stop bleeding with gauze or silver nitrate sticks
- Remove speculum.

AFTER THE PROCEDURE

- If needed, specimens may be sent to pathology for examination
- RhoGAM may be needed within 72 hours following procedure if patient has Rh negative blood type
- Observe patient after procedure to rule out hemorrhage
- Consider prophylactic antibiotics.

SELF-ASSESSMENT QUIZ

1. Dilatation and curettage is traditionally performed as:
    a. Ultrasound-guided procedure
    b. Fluoroscopy-guided procedure
    c. Blind procedure
    d. Hysterocopy-guided procedure
    e. None of the above
2. Dilatation and curettage is
    a. A diagnostic procedure
    b. A therapeutic procedure
    c. Diagnostic and therapeutic procedure
    d. None of the above
3. In patients with cervical stenosis in whom uterine sounding and cervical dilatation with dilators cannot be achieved, the ease of dilatation may be enhanced with
    a. Laminaria
    b. Vaginal misoprostol
    c. All of the above
    d. None of the above

Contd...

Contd...

4. Curettage is performed
    a. From the fundus to the internal cervical os
    b. The tissue is removed with a curette through the external cervical os
    c. The tissue removed from the uterine cavity is collected for pathology assessment
    d. All of the above
    e. None of the above
5. Indications for a diagnostic dilatation and curettage are:
    a. 1st trimester pregnancy
    b. Retained products of conception
    c. 2nd and 3rd trimester pregnancy
    d. Abnormal uterine bleeding
    e. a + c
    f. b + d

Answers

1. c   2. c   3. c   4. d   5. f

SUGGESTED READING

1. Demirkiran F, Yavuz E, Erenel H, Bese T, Arvas M, Sanioglu C. Which is the best technique for endometrial sampling? Aspiration (pipelle) versus dilatation and curettage (D&C). Arch Gynecol Obstet. 2012;286(5):1277-82.
2. Dysfunctional Uterine Bleeding. In: Emons SJ. Pediatric and Adolescent Gynecology. 5th ed. Philadelphia: Lippincott Williams & Wilkins; 2004.
3. Glantz JC, Shomento S. Comparison of paracervical block techniques during first trimester preganancy termination. International J Gynecol Obstet. 2001;72(2):171-8.
4. Mankowski JL, Klingston J, Moran T, Nager CW, Lukacz ES. Paracervical compared with intracervical lidocaine for suction curettage: a randomized controlled trial. Obstet Gynecol. 2009;113(5):1052-7.
5. Rock JA, Jones HW. Surgery for Benign Gynecologic Conditions. In: Telinde's Operative Gynecology. 10th ed. Philadelphia, PA: Lippincott Williams & Wilkins; 2008:598-605;784-7.
6. Wheeless CR, Roennburg ML. Suction Curettage for Abortion. Atlas of Pelvic Surgery Online Edition. Available at http://www.atlasofpelvicsurgery.com/5Uterus/2SuctionCurettageandAbortion/chap5sec2.html; Accessed July, 2014.

Intrauterine Device Placement and Removal

Mendez MD, Kupesic Plavsic S

INTRODUCTION/BACKGROUND

- An intrauterine device is a long-term yet reversible method of birth control
  - The hormone (progestin) releasing device can stay in place for 5 years
  - The copper coated IUD can stay in place for 10 years
- A good candidate for this device will be a woman who has already given birth and is in a monogamous relationship.

UNIVERSAL PRECAUTIONS

- Gloves must be worn while placing IUD
- Evaluate the need for face and eye protection as well as a gown.

OBTAIN INFORMED CONSENT

- Introduce yourself to the patient
- Explain the procedure to the patient, as well as the risks and benefits
- Gain informed consent to continue.

INDICATIONS

- Birth control
- Anemia (for hormone-releasing IUD)
- Menorrhagia (for hormone-releasing IUD)
- Dysmenorrhea (for hormone-releasing IUD).

CONTRAINDICATIONS

- **Pregnancy**
- History of pelvic inflammatory disease
- Uterine abnormality
- **Untreated** cervicitis
- Genital actinomycosis
- **Copper:** Wilson's disease or copper allergy
- Hormone releasing: Breast carcinoma, liver disease or allergy to levonorgestrel.

COMPLICATIONS

- Infection
- Bleeding
- Pain
- Uterine perforation.

BASIC EQUIPMENT

- Sterile and nonsterile gloves
- Sterile vaginal speculum with sterile gel
- Iodine swabs, ring forceps and 4 × 4 gauze
- Cervical tenaculum
- Sterile scissors
- Sterile IUD package
- Uterine sound
- Have cervical dilators available.

SITES/POSITIONING

- The patient should be positioned supine in the dorsal lithotomy position.

PREPARATION

- An nonsteroidal anti-inflammatory drug (NSAID) may be given to the patient 1 hour prior to IUD insertion
- Through the sterile packing, fold the IUD arms into the insertion tube
- With nonsterile gloves, perform bimanual examination to check uterine angulation, size and shape
- Insert speculum and clean cervix using forceps and cotton soaked with iodine.

PROCEDURE STEPS

- Don sterile gloves and place tenaculum on the anterior lip of the cervix
  - Hold light retraction

- Insert the uterine sound through the cervical os
  - Average lengths are 6–8 cm
  - If sound is not advancing, consider cervical dilators
- Place the insertion rod into insertion tube
- Insert the IUD through the cervical os to the depth sounded
  - Withdraw the inner rod 2 cm to spread the IUD arms
  - Remove the insertion tube
- Trim threads to 3 cm with the sterile scissors and remove the tenaculum
- Hold pressure with gauze held in forceps if the tenaculum sites are bleeding.

REMOVAL

- The hormone-eluting IUD should be removed in 5 years and the copper IUD within 10 years
- Grasp the strings with forceps and remove IUD with a gentle retracting pressure
  - The patient may experience some bleeding or cramping.

SELF-ASSESSMENT QUIZ

1. The most common side-effects of copper IUD are:
   a. Increase in menstrual blood loss   b. Dysmenorrhea
   c. High failure rate   d. a + b
   e. b + c
2. The benefits of using progestin releasing IUD are:
   a. Reduced menorrhagia   b. Reduced dysmenorrhea
   c. a +b   d. b + c
3. Contraindications for IUD use are:
   a. Pregnancy   b. Unexplained vaginal bleeding
   c. Multiple sexual partners   d. All of the above
   e. None of the above
4. Most common complications of IUD insertion include:
   a. Uterine fibroid   b. Uterine cramping
   c. Cervical polyp   d. Endometrial hyperplasia
5. Choose the most accurate option:
   a. IUD is a permanent contraception   b. IUD is a reversible contraception
   c. Can be used in nulliparous patients   d. Cannot be used in nulliparous patients
   e. a + c   f. b + c
   g. b + d

Answers

1. d   2. c   3. d   4. b   5. f

SUGGESTED READING

1. American College of Obstetricians and Gynecologists. ACOG Practice Bulletin No. 121: Long-acting reversible contraception: Implants and intrauterine devices. Obstet Gynecol. 2011;118:184.

2. Committee on Adolescent Health Care Long-Acting Reversible Contraception Working Group, The American College of Obstetricians and Gynecologists. Committee opinion no. 539: adolescents and long-acting reversible contraception: implants and intrauterine devices. Obstet Gynecol. 2012;120:983.

3. Grimes DA, Schulz KF. Antibiotic prophylaxis for intrauterine contraceptive device insertion. Cochrane Database Syst Rev. 2001;CD001327.

4. Johnson BA. Insertion and Removal of Intrauterine Devices. Am Fam Physician. 2005;71(1)95-102.

5. Mirena levonorgestrel-releasing intrauterine system: Physician package insert. Montville, NJ: Berlex Laboratories; 2003.

6. Nelson AL. The intrauterine contraceptive device. Obstet Gynecol Clin North Am. 2000;27:723-40.

7. Paragard T380A intrauterine copper contraceptive: Prescribing information and instructions for use, Tonawanda, NJ: FEI Products; 2003.

8. US Selected Practice Recommendations for Contraceptive Use, 2013. http://www.cdc.gov/mmwr/pdf/rr/rr62e0614.pdf. Accessed July. 14 2014.

Index